25 Natural Ways to Relieve PMS

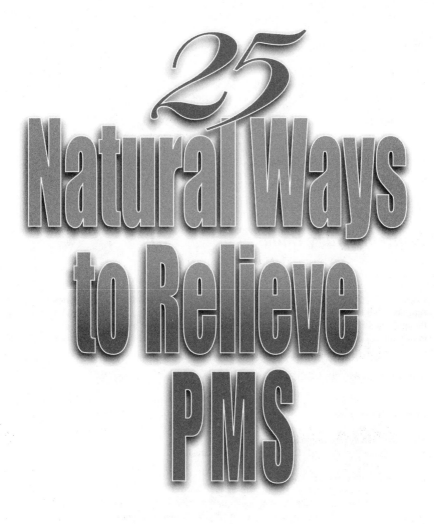

25 Natural Ways to Relieve PMS

NADINE TAYLOR, M.S., R.D.

Contemporary Books

Chicago New York San Francisco Lisbon London Madrid Mexico City
Milan New Delhi San Juan Seoul Singapore Sydney Toronto

Library of Congress Cataloging-in-Publication Data

Taylor, Nadine.
    25 natural ways to relieve PMS / Nadine Taylor.
        p.   cm.   (25 natural ways . . . series)
    Includes index.
    ISBN 0-658-01376-9
    1. Menopause—Complications—Alternative treatment.   2. Premenstrual
syndrome—Alternative treatment.   I. Title: Twenty-five natural ways to relieve
PMS. II. Title. III. Series.

RG165 .T39   2002
618.1'72—dc21   2001050251

Contemporary Books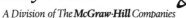

A Division of The McGraw·Hill Companies

2 3 4 5 6 7 8 9 0 DOC/DOC 1 0 9 8 7 6 5 4 3 2

ISBN 0-658-01376-9

This book was set in Garamond
Printed and bound by R. R. Donnelley—Crawfordsville

Cover design by Jeanette Wojtyla

McGraw-Hill books are available at special quantity discounts to use as premiums and
sales promotions, or for use in corporate training programs. For more information, please
write to the Director of Special Sales, Professional Publishing, McGraw-Hill, Two Penn
Plaza, New York, NY 10121-2298. Or contact your local bookstore.

The purpose of this book is to educate. It is sold with the understanding that the publisher
and author shall have neither liability nor responsibility for any injury caused or alleged to
be caused directly or indirectly by the information contained in this book. While every
effort has been made to ensure its accuracy, the book's contents should not be construed
as medical advice. Each person's health needs are unique. To obtain recommendations
appropriate to your particular situation, please consult a health care provider.

This book is printed on acid-free paper.

For my three nieces—Kristen, Melanie, and Heather.
Here's hoping you'll never need this book!

Contents

Introduction

Oh boy, here it comes again! At the age of thirty-seven, I've gone through this process so many times I don't even have to look at the calendar to know that my period will be arriving in just about . . . oh, I'd say five days. There are plenty of signs heralding the approach of my monthly "visitor"—but the main one is that I get furious at the drop of a hat! (Sure enough, I had a big fight with my husband Barry this morning about . . . what was it about anyway? Something silly, I know that much.) Then there's the puffy stomach and its twin companions: swollen, tender breasts. I often find myself getting depressed for no real reason at this time of the month and *always* develop a voracious appetite for sweets. (WHY is there no chocolate in this house?!) Other than the fact that PMS disrupts my life for a few days each month, it's not such a big problem for me. At least it doesn't give me migraines, like it does my friend Melinda, who is laid out flat for at least three days every fourth week.

Does any of this sound familiar? Probably, since as many as forty million women suffer regularly from these and other symptoms, collectively known as Premenstrual Syndrome, or PMS. It's been estimated that 85 percent of women in their childbearing years experience some of the symptoms of PMS at least once in a while, 40 percent get

PMS regularly, and 10 to 15 percent suffer from severe symptoms that seriously upset their lives. The symptoms of PMS, which can be both physical and psychological, appear between one and fourteen days prior to menstruation and then, as if by magic, disappear once the menstrual period actually begins. Typically the woman is then symptom-free for the next two to three weeks, before the whole process is repeated.

A cornucopia of some one hundred to two hundred symptoms have been attributed to PMS, but the most common include:

Acne
Aggressiveness
Anxiety
Backaches
Binge eating
Bloating
Breast tenderness and/or swelling
Cravings for sweets
Crying easily
Depression
Dizziness
Fatigue
Headaches, including migraines
Hostility
Irritability
Joint pain
Memory loss
Mood swings
Thirst
Weight gain

Other less common (but very real) PMS symptoms are constipation, asthma, disorientation, diarrhea, drug abuse, heaviness of the legs, hypersensitivity to sound, self-inflicted injuries, shakiness, and suicidal thoughts, among others. How delightful—especially if you have to go through it once a month! Some researchers have also found that those with severe PMS are more likely to indulge in extreme behavior during this time, such as drug and alcohol abuse, violent crime, accidents—you get the idea.

Luckily, *nobody* suffers from all of these symptoms, but even a single one can be too much if it recurs twelve times a year. PMS can wreak havoc on just about every area of a woman's life—work, family, friends, and peace of mind. My friend Jane misses work two or three days a month because of PMS-related dizziness, fatigue, and depression. "It simply wipes me out," she says. "I can't function at all during those few days, so I just stay home and try to sleep it off." Robin, a coworker of mine, told me that her monthly mood swings were wrecking her home life. "Once I get through 'PMS-ing,' I spend the next week or two running around trying to clean up the messes I've made in my relationships. But by the time everybody's forgiven and forgotten, I'm off on another cycle." Another friend, Denise, confided, "I get so tired of feeling lousy during that week before my period that I'm actually glad once the darn thing finally starts. Even though I get terrible cramps, it's better than feeling depressed, bloated, and ticked off all the time."

HOW DO YOU KNOW IF YOU'VE GOT PMS?

Up until recently, many doctors and other experts insisted that PMS didn't really exist. It was "all in your mind," they said. So, many women who really suffered from this disorder were led to believe they were self-indulgent, hypersensitive, or just plain crazy. Today, thank goodness, PMS is accepted as a true disorder or disease. But the pendulum may have swung too far, because almost every woman complains about PMS when she may, in fact, *not* have it. For example, the lower back pain and any other discomforts experienced *during* the menstrual period are not symptoms of PMS. And certain well-known symptoms of PMS may quite possibly be signs of something entirely different. For example, it's easy to mistake your depression over a lost job or failing marriage for the depression of PMS; or to attribute your lower back pain and craving for sweets to PMS when they may actually be signs of bad posture and hypoglycemia. That's why it's important that you discuss your symptoms with your doctor and get a thorough check-up to rule out other causes of your physical or psychological distress. In the meantime, remember that there are three major hallmarks of PMS:

- The symptoms appear within two weeks before the onset of your period.
- You're getting symptoms all month, but they're markedly *worse* during the week or so before your period.
- The symptoms clear up once your period begins or a couple of days into it.

KEEP AN ACCOUNT OF YOUR SYMPTOMS

The best way—and only way—to be sure that you're experiencing true PMS is to keep an account of your symptoms. Each day, using a diary or a calendar, make a note of any physical or psychological disturbances you experience (headache, depression, etc.) and rank them according to severity. I like to use 1 for mild, 2 for moderate, and 3 for severe. Be sure to mark the days of your menstrual period, as well. Do this for at least two months, then look for a pattern. Do your symptoms seem to be more frequent and/or severe during the week or so before your period? If so, they're probably due to PMS. If, on the other hand, you're getting symptoms throughout the month and they don't seem to get worse during the premenstrual phase, something else is likely to be the cause.

THE DEBUT OF PMS

PMS typically makes its first appearance in conjunction with one of the "Three P's"—at puberty, after a first pregnancy, or when starting or stopping the pill (oral contraceptives). It tends to get worse with pregnancy and with age, and may get steadily worse until menopause, when symptoms fall off (usually around the age of fifty). But surgically-induced menopause (hysterectomy) is *rarely* a cure for PMS. A women who has had her uterus and/or ovaries removed prior to menopause sometimes continues to experience symptoms of PMS until she reaches the typical age of menopause. Evidently, the body continues to go through hormonal cycles whether your organs are intact or not!

THE MYSTICAL, MEANDERING MENSTRUAL CYCLE

To understand the origins of PMS, you need to know a few basics about the menstrual cycle. A "typical" menstrual cycle lasts for twenty-eight days (four weeks), with Day One being the first day of menstruation. The cycle is directed by the rise and fall of two hormones, estrogen and progesterone, each of which follows its own cycle.

The whole process begins in the hypothalamus, a sort of "glandular control center" in the brain. The hypothalamus triggers the menstrual cycle by telling the pituitary gland to produce a hormone called *follicle-stimulating hormone* (FSH), which then travels to the ovaries. At birth, the ovaries already contain all of the eggs a woman will ever have, each of which lies quietly in a dormant state encased in a covering called a *follicle*. But the follicle is more than just a protective coating. When FSH makes its monthly trip to the ovaries, the follicles suddenly begin to grow. At the same time, they become hormone-producing machines, pumping out a very important product called *estrogen.* Estrogen stimulates the thickening of the uterine lining and the growth of uterine blood vessels to prepare a soft, nutrient-rich place for a fertilized egg to lodge—just in case a pregnancy should occur this month. As the follicles increase in size, they produce greater and greater amounts of estrogen. But one follicle outgrows all the others (sort of like a queen bee), and this follicle is the one that will produce this month's egg.

When the estrogen levels reach a peak (around Day Fourteen), the pituitary gland slows down its production of FSH, which results in a slight dip in estrogen levels. At the same time, the pituitary gland increases production of a different hormone called *luteinizing hormone* (LH). The combination of the drop in FSH and the rise in LH causes the mature egg to pop out of its follicle and set sail on a three- to four-day voyage down the fallopian tube toward the uterus. If the egg should encounter sperm during this short journey, it may become fertilized.

Meanwhile, the egg's discarded home, the follicle (now called the *corpus luteum*) still has work to do. It continues to make estrogen, but also begins to manufacture the hormone *progesterone.* Progesterone makes the uterine lining spongy, working in tandem with estrogen to make preparations for a possible pregnancy. On or near Day Twenty-Three, the levels of both hormones reach an all-time high. If, however, the egg hasn't been fertilized, all bets are off. During the next five days, both estrogen and progesterone levels will drop sharply, causing the uterus to break down its newly-thickened lining and shed it. The process of discharging the lining (menstruation) begins about five days after the estrogen-progesterone peak and is counted as Day One of a new menstrual cycle. To help shed the lining, the body releases hormone-like substances called *prostaglandins,* which stimulate the contraction of the uterus (menstrual cramps).

So, hormonally speaking, we have two completely different cycles taking place, one involving estrogen, the other progesterone. Both begin at very low levels on Day One and end at very low levels on Day Twenty-Eight. But in between there are major differences: estrogen levels climb from next to nothing on Day One to a peak just before ovulation (Day Fourteen), when they dip for a few days, but not all the way down to baseline level. Then they continue to rise, reaching a second peak about five days before menstruation (Day Twenty-Three) before taking a major dive and plummeting all the way back down to baseline by Day Twenty-Eight, thus triggering menstruation. Progesterone levels, on the other hand, stay at baseline for the first half of the cycle (until ovulation on or near Day Fourteen), then they begin to rise, reaching their peak at the same time that estrogen levels reach their second peak (Day Twenty-Three). Like estrogen, progesterone levels drop off sharply after Day Twenty-Three, returning to baseline by Day Twenty-Eight when menstruation begins.

SO WHAT DO THESE HORMONE CYCLES HAVE TO DO WITH PMS?

Hormones are extremely powerful substances, so any discrepancy in the amount that's manufactured or the timing of the release is bound to make a major difference in the way your body functions and how you feel. Although the theories regarding the origins of PMS are just that—theories—many experts believe that hormonal fluctuations or imbalances are the major culprits. It's quite possible that your PMS could be due to one or more of the following:

• **The sudden drop in hormone levels**—When estrogen and progesterone levels take a nosedive around Day Twenty-Three, many women experience PMS symptoms. Those who experience menstrual migraines are much more likely to get one at this time. The drop in estrogen levels that occurs with ovulation (Day Fourteen) can also trigger symptoms in a few women, although they are usually less severe than those occurring shortly before the menstrual period.

• **Estrogen levels that are too high**—Estrogen promotes water retention, so excessive amounts of this hormone are probably the cause of the weight gain, tissue swelling, bloating, and breast tenderness seen with PMS. Excess estrogen can also bring about anxiety, depression, emotional hypersensitivity, fatigue, low blood sugar, migraine headaches, and sleeplessness, all symptoms of PMS. In addition, too much estrogen can cause magnesium deficiency, which may contribute to sugar cravings and mood swings. An excess of estrogen can result from poor diet, stress, too much body fat (fatty tissue produces estrogen), estrogen-only hormone replacement therapy, oral contraceptives, or liver dysfunction. (The liver deactivates old estrogen once it's done its job, so if that organ is not working well, estrogen levels can build up.) And we're constantly exposed to pseudo-estrogens through industrial wastes, hormone-laden meats, pesticides, plastics, various furnishings, and even soaps, all of which can drive up our bodily estrogen levels.

• **Progesterone levels that are too low**—Progesterone acts as a counterbalance to estrogen, so if you've got too little progesterone, the symptoms of estrogen excess may appear—even if your estrogen levels are normal. Progesterone plays several important roles in the body. It acts as a natural diuretic, helps the body break down and use fat for energy, stabilizes blood sugar levels, has an antidepressant effect, and helps you sleep, among other things. Without enough progesterone, you may experience the opposite effects. (Hmmm—sounds like PMS to me!) A lack of progesterone can be due to the presence of too much estrogen or may result from other conditions such as menopause (which causes progesterone levels to sink nearly to zero) or the lack of ovulation. (Remember, it's the old discarded home of the egg—the follicle—that manufactures progesterone, once the egg begins its journey through the fallopian tube. And yes, you can have your period even if you haven't ovulated.) Diet may also play a part in depleted progesterone levels. Too much animal fat often interferes with the manufacture of progesterone, as can deficiencies in beta-carotene and/or vitamin E. Finally, stress may lower progesterone levels because it triggers the release of large amounts of the hormone *cortisol,* which competes with progesterone for common receptor sites.

• **Estrogen levels that are too low**—Even though too much estrogen can be a problem, you don't want your levels of this hormone to fall too low, either. Estrogen plays an important role in fighting depression by stimulating the brain cells that respond to the hormone *serotonin*. Often described as the "feel good" hormone, serotonin exerts tranquilizing and mood-enhancing effects on the brain. A lack of serotonin results in plenty of unpleasant side effects, including depression, irritability, increased sensitivity to pain, migraine headaches, hot flashes, night sweats, and vaginal dryness. Low levels of estrogen may result from menopause, anorexia, excessive exercise, stress, poor diet, and cigarette smoking, among other things.

OTHER POSSIBLE CAUSES OF PMS

But hormones aren't the only monkey wrench in the machinery. Plenty of other things appear to contribute to the appearance of PMS and its severity, including:

• **Heredity**—Yes, unfortunately if your mother, your aunt, and your sister all have PMS, you're likely to suffer from it, too.

• **Birth control pills**—"The pill" seems to cut both ways. That is, in some people it can bring on PMS or make an existing case worse, while in others it makes PMS recede, depending upon whether it evens out your hormones or causes an imbalance.

• **Poor dietary habits**—What you eat can make PMS worse, especially if you take in high amounts of caffeine, alcohol, sugar, salt, or saturated fat. And deficiencies in certain nutrients can compound the trouble. PMS symptoms get worse if you have low levels of vitamin A (and its plant form, beta-carotene), vitamins B_6 and B_{12}, choline, vitamins C and E, calcium, magnesium, potassium, and/or zinc.

• **Irregularities in certain brain chemicals** called *neurotransmitters* may also bring on PMS, causing an imbalance in hormone production, the retention of water, and alterations in mood and behavior. Insufficient amounts of the neurotransmitter serotonin, as noted earlier, may be responsible for increased anxiety, irritability, and insomnia.

Other possible causes of PMS include a lack of exercise, stress, malfunction of the thyroid gland, yeast overgrowth, food allergies, mercury fillings, and even parasites—but the truth is, no one really knows for sure. Experts *do* seem to agree, however, that PMS is most often brought on by hormonal imbalances, fluid retention, vitamin deficiencies, and/or low blood sugar.

RISK FACTORS FOR PMS

Ever wonder why you have PMS but your best friend sails through with nary a symptom? It could be due to the cards you've been dealt in life, but it's probably also due to the way you're playing them. Still, certain factors will increase your chances of getting PMS:

- Your mother, aunt, grandmother, or sister has it.
- You have children (PMS tends to get worse with each child).
- You're over thirty (PMS hits hardest when you're in your thirties and forties).
- You've had trouble tolerating the birth control pill.
- You've suffered from toxemia while pregnant.
- You don't exercise.
- You're significantly stressed.
- Your dietary habits are poor.
- Your weight tends to go up and down.

OKAY, SO I'VE GOT PMS. NOW WHAT?

While you can't change the fact that, say, you're over thirty, you have three kids, and the birth control pill makes you crazy, you *can* do something about your diet, the amount of exercise you get, your weight, and your stress levels. Researchers have found that making positive changes in these areas can make a decided difference in how many PMS symptoms you experience and how severe they are. And when you think about it, it makes sense. Let's face facts: we live unnatural, highly-stressed, complicated lives that have very little in common with our ancestor, the cave woman. Yet our bodies are remarkably similar to hers in design. Is it any wonder that our body equilibrium gets thrown out of whack when we're stuffed with high-fat, low-nutrient foods, stuck in chairs for the major part of our days, and loaded with stress that we passively absorb?

The good news is that PMS is not a figment of your imagination, and you *can* do something about it. By following a few simple dietary changes, getting more exercise, and using the other completely natural, safe, and—surprise!—enjoyable methods outlined in this book, you may be able to decrease or even eliminate many of your most prominent symptoms. You really don't have to suffer any longer. Finally, instead of putting everything on hold for up to two weeks every month, you can start living life to the fullest every single day!

1

Eat Wisely and Well

Okay, I admit it. There's a whole lot of confusion surrounding PMS; its origins, symptoms, and treatments all seem to be a bit hazy, at best. But there's one thing the experts do agree on—changing your diet almost always works to your advantage. That is, changing your diet to one based primarily on whole grains; fresh, organic vegetables and fruits; legumes; nuts; seeds; and smaller amounts of fish, chicken, and nonfat dairy products. This is one of the absolute best things you can do to ward off many of the major PMS symptoms, including mood swings, depression, anxiety, lethargy, aggression, binge eating, weight gain, and headache. And why wouldn't it be? If your body seems to be off-kilter (a pretty fair description of PMS), fueling it with plenty of high-quality, nutrient-dense foods seems like an obvious ticket to getting it back on track.

Yet there's more to the PMS-diet connection than that. For example, eating certain foods can increase the inflammation response (leading to migraine headaches, among other things), while eating other foods can decrease inflammation. Similarly, water retention is made worse by some foods, yet eased by others. Some foods contribute to hormone imbalances, while others help restore balance. High-sugar foods (including fruit that's eaten by itself) can send your blood sugar soaring at first, then crashing down, bringing along intense irritabil-

1

ity, dizziness, fatigue, or aggression. And some foods can make you anxious, while their counterparts soothe you.

Compared to women who don't have PMS, those who do have this condition generally take in more sugar, refined carbohydrates, dairy products, and sodium but less iron, zinc, and manganese. It seems clear that what you eat—and what you don't eat—can make a major difference in the way your body responds, particularly during the PMS phase of your monthly cycle. So the very first thing you should do in your quest to stamp out PMS is look to your diet and see where you can make positive changes.

Diet is such an integral part of PMS control that I decided to devote the first ten chapters of this book to its various aspects. But to get the ball rolling, let's begin with a look at the elements of the good old, high-nutrient, low-fat diet—the mainstay of good health. I hope you don't shudder when you read the word *diet*. What we're discussing in this chapter is simply how to eat well, with the goal of making your body as healthy and full of life as possible. This is *not* intended to be a weight loss plan or to deprive you in any way. It's just to remind you about the kinds of foods that can nourish your body, as opposed to the processed, preservative-laden, fatty foods most of us tend to rely on these days. So go ahead—eat up! Just make sure you're filling your body with highly nutritious foods instead of junk! I guarantee that once you start eating wisely and well, you'll feel so good you'll never want to return to your old bad habits.

WHAT MAKES UP A HEALTHY DIET?

Okay, there's a short answer to this and a long one. For those of you who like to get to the point and move on, the short answer is this:

- Eat all the fresh vegetables, fruits, whole grains, and legumes (dried beans, peas, etc.) that you want.

- Limit your intake of low-fiber foods made from refined grains (white bread, pasta, white rice, cake, cookies, etc.).
- Eat small amounts of lean meat, fish, or poultry as a protein source (a total of about 5–7 oz. cooked per day). Legumes (dried beans, peas, or nuts) can be substituted as a source of protein (1–1½ cup cooked beans or peas or ½–1 cup nuts = 1 serving). Eggs are also okay (1 serving = 2 eggs), but limit your eggs to three a week.
- Don't eat fried foods or foods cooked in more than 1–2 tsp. oil.
- Limit added fats to 1–2 T. per day and avoid saturated fats (butter, animal fat, etc.)
- Eat or drink two to three servings of nonfat dairy products.
- Drink at least eight glasses of water per day.

If you stick to these dietary guidelines, you should be getting just about everything your body needs to maintain good health—and your nutrient status will be a lot better than that of the average person.

Now for the longer, more complex answer to "What makes up a healthy diet?" Each of the following food groups makes unique contributions to a healthy diet that aren't supplied in sufficient quantities by any other group. So if you don't get enough servings from each of these groups, your nutrient status will suffer. That's why the U.S. Department of Agriculture came up with a system of classifying foods and has recommended eating a certain number of servings from each group to ensure optimal health. But besides all that, each group provides special nutrients that can help ease your PMS symptoms. That should give you extra incentive to pay close attention to what you eat! Check out the following and see what each group can do for you.

Bread, Cereal, Rice, Pasta—Six to Eleven Servings

Serving size: One piece of bread, ½ cup cooked rice or pasta, 1 oz. ready to eat cereal

Why this group is important: Whole-grain versions of these foods provide good amounts of fiber, carbohydrates, B vitamins, vitamin E, magnesium, iron, and zinc.

What this group does to combat PMS: The B vitamins found in the Bread, Cereal, Rice, and Pasta group work to stabilize brain chemistry, regulate glucose metabolism, and inactivate "old" estrogen in the liver. Vitamin B_6 helps ease many PMS symptoms, including irritability, mood swings, fatigue, fluid retention, sugar craving, and breast tenderness. Fiber helps to stabilize blood sugar, which tends to become more erratic during the PMS phase. Vitamin E helps reduce breast tenderness, sugar cravings, depression, irritability, and anxiety. Magnesium helps ease menstrual migraines, PMS-related sugar cravings, fatigue, and mood swings, while normalizing glucose metabolism and aiding in the absorption of calcium, a natural tranquilizer. Zinc stabilizes the mood, controls acne, and helps keep estrogen levels in balance.

NOTE: Look for the "brown variety" when you're shopping—brown rice, whole wheat, whole oats, etc.—and skip the white stuff.

Green Leafy Vegetables, Yellow-Orange Fruits and Vegetables—At Least Three Servings

Serving size: One serving = one medium-sized fruit or vegetable; ½ cup cooked; 1 cup (chopped) raw; ½ cup juice

Why this group is important: Green, leafy veggies are great sources of folic acid, magnesium, and vitamin C, while yellow-orange fruits and vegetables provide good amounts of beta-carotene and potassium.

What this group does to combat PMS: Vitamin C is necessary for the synthesis of *adrenocorticotropin* (the hormone that triggers the release of estrogen and progesterone). The acne and other skin disorders that erupt during the PMS phase might be eased by beta-carotene or zinc. Potassium can help fight fatigue, while fruits and vegetables containing high amounts of water (think watermelon, watercress, cucumbers, cantaloupe, etc.) may decrease water retention.

NOTE: Eat your vegetables and fruits raw—or very lightly cooked—whenever possible. Although fruit and vegetable juices provide vitamins and minerals, they've been stripped of their fiber, so juice should make up only one serving per day.

Other Vegetables and Fruits—At Least Two Servings

Serving size: One medium-sized fruit or vegetable; ½ cup cooked; 1 cup (chopped) raw; ½ cup juice

Why this group is important: Vegetables and fruits in general are good sources of carbohydrate, fiber, vitamin C, beta-carotene, folic acid, magnesium, and potassium.

What this group does to combat PMS: Fiber aids in regulation of blood sugar levels, while magnesium may help ease headaches, bloating, weight gain, and breast tenderness. Folic acid helps prevent anemia, which can bring on fatigue that could be mistaken for a symptom of PMS.

NOTE: Same recommendations apply as for green leafies and yellow-orange fruits and vegetables. Also, try to make sure at least one serving is rich in vitamin C (e.g., citrus, broccoli, berries, cantaloupe, kiwi, etc.).

Lean Meat, Poultry, Fish, Eggs, Soy, Nuts, Legumes—Two to Three Servings

Serving size: 2–3 oz. cooked lean meat, fish, or poultry (for a total of 5–7 oz. per day), two eggs, ½ cup tofu or soybeans, 4 T. peanut butter, ½–1 cup nuts, 1 cup cooked legumes

Why this group is important: This group is your major source of protein, but also offers B vitamins, folic acid, phosphorus, magnesium, iron, and zinc. Vegetarian protein is preferred since it raises the body's levels of B_6 and magnesium and helps reduce excess estrogen, all of which are helpful for controlling PMS symptoms.

What this group does to combat PMS: Fish that contain omega-3 fatty acids (salmon, mackerel, Atlantic sturgeon, herring, etc.—see Chapter 7) help reduce the inflammation response, lessen breast tenderness, and ease menstrual cramps. Protein in general helps to stabilize the blood sugar, preventing the dip in blood glucose that can bring about depression, fatigue, and irritability. And the iron present in most protein sources helps prevent anemia and its resulting fatigue. In addition, soy-based foods are an excellent source of plant estrogens, which help relieve PMS by competing with your own estrogen for receptor sites. Since less of your own estrogen can be "activated" when plant estrogen crowds it out, excessively high levels of estrogen may recede.

NOTE: Emphasize vegetable protein and fish that contain omega-3 fatty acids, and limit your eggs to three per week, since they contain saturated fat, which can increase symptoms of PMS. If you do eat meat and/or poultry, buy the hormone-free variety (available at health food stores) to avoid a buildup of estrogen in your body. Also trim the fat off before cooking, since saturated fat (animal fat) increases production of the hormone *prostaglandin*, which can lead to lowered levels of progesterone and an increase in bloating, cramping, and mood swings.

Milk, Yogurt, Cheese—Two to Three Servings

Serving size: 1 cup milk or yogurt, 1 oz. cheese, or 3 oz. canned mackerel, salmon, or sardines eaten *with* the bones.

Why this group is important: The major contributions of this group are calcium, magnesium, phosphorus, carbohydrate, protein, riboflavin, vitamin D, and zinc. Calcium, of course, is of vital importance in the maintenance of healthy bones and prevention of osteoporosis.

What this group does to combat PMS: Calcium and magnesium, in particular, have been found to be helpful in treating PMS symptoms. Calcium may relieve irritability, depression, and mood swings, while magnesium may help ease headaches, bloating, weight gain, and breast tenderness.

NOTE: Don't overdo it on the dairy products. They typically have a high sodium content (even milk!), which means they can exacerbate water retention. The saturated fat contained in whole milk and full-fat cheeses can increase estrogen levels and help produce the kind of prostaglandins that increase cramping, bloating, and mood swings. Limit your consumption of dairy products to two or three servings of the nonfat variety. Also, yogurt should be plain, not sweetened with sugar or artificial sweeteners. If dairy products seem to make your PMS worse, try soy milk, leafy green vegetables, almonds, or other sources of calcium and be sure to take a calcium supplement.

Now that I've laid out what you should be eating and how much, you're probably saying, "Wow, that's a lot of food! I could never eat that much." It *is* a lot of food—or it can be if you eat the maximum amount of servings—but you'll probably find that you've got room for at least the minimum number of servings once you cut back on high-sugar, high-fat foods. Snack foods, desserts, fried foods, and the like tend to fill you up but provide little nutritional value. So limit them—or, even better, eliminate them—and don't waste your appetite on junk. Make every bite count. Not only will this help lessen your PMS symptoms, it will improve your energy level, your resistance to disease, and your overall health.

EAT SEVERAL SMALL MEALS PER DAY

Eating a wide variety of the most nutrient-dense foods you can find, spread throughout the day in five to six small meals, is probably the number-one most effective way of combating premenstrual irritability, aggression, fatigue, weakness, headaches, shakiness, and dizziness. That's because these problems are often caused by low blood sugar, a problem that may rear its ugly head a week or so before the arrival of the menstrual period. Changes in body chemistry during that time make your body more responsive to *insulin*, the hormone that helps glucose in the bloodstream enter the body's cells, where it's used for food.

But during the week before your period, insulin often starts working a little "too well," which leaves you with lower than normal levels of blood glucose, or *hypoglycemia*. That's when you start getting shaky, fatigued, hungry, and irritable—the same way you might feel if you have to wait too long for lunch. But you can combat this condition by eating regularly throughout the day to keep blood glucose at a fairly even level. Just keep these frequent meals on the small side (unless you're in the market for a weight gain) and make sure each one includes a protein-rich food (legumes, cottage cheese, eggs, nuts, lean meat, poultry, etc.) and a high-fiber food (whole grains, vegetables, fruits, etc.). Both protein and fiber help slow the entrance of glucose into the cells, so your meal doesn't result in a sudden jump in blood glucose followed by a big drop once the insulin goes into action. Instead, blood glucose levels gradually rise and fall as each meal is eaten and digested. Before your glucose levels reach uncomfortably low points, you'll eat another meal, and your glucose will again be on the rise.

Just a couple of hard-and-fast rules:

- Don't skip meals.
- Don't fast.
- Don't eat sugary snacks (including fruit) without also eating something containing protein and fiber.
- Do eat as soon as you feel hungry, weak, faint, irritable, or show any other signs of hypoglycemia.
- Do eat enough to satisfy yourself.

A DAY IN THE LIFE OF "THE PMS DIET"

Here's what one nutrient-packed day of "The PMS Diet" might look like:

Breakfast

1 oz. whole-grain oatmeal, cooked
1 piece whole-wheat toast w/soy margarine
⅓ cup nonfat cottage cheese
1 fresh nectarine

Mid-morning Snack/Meal

1 oz. whole-grain crackers
1 oz. sardines packed in water (eaten with the bones)

Lunch

1 piece whole-wheat bread
1–2 cups split pea soup
Salad made with 1 cup spinach leaves, ½ grated carrot, ½ tomato
Dressing made with olive oil

Mid-afternoon Snack/Meal

1 whole-wheat bran muffin
1 cup nonfat yogurt

Dinner

3 oz. broiled salmon
½ cup brown rice
1 cup steamed broccoli
½ cantaloupe with ½ cup berries

Evening Snack/Meal

½ cup toasted soy nuts
1 fresh peach

STAY AWAY FROM CASS

Even if you do nothing else, chances are excellent that you can decrease your PMS symptoms just by eliminating four things from your diet:

- Caffeine
- Alcohol
- Sugar
- Salt

These four dietary demons, which I've nicknamed CASS for convenience, increase the body's toxic load and put plenty of stress on the system, both of which can interfere with the body's ability to achieve and maintain balance. An overload of toxins may also slow the processing of estrogen and/or progesterone. That's because the liver, the body's major detoxifying organ, is also in charge of breaking down and disposing of hormones. Eating too many "stressful" foods can overwork the liver and make it less effective overall, allowing hormones to build up or become imbalanced. So give your liver—and the rest of your body—a break! Cut back on CASS and discover how much better you can feel. (For more on CASS and its PMS-inducing tricks, see Chapters 2, 3, 4, and 5.)

HELLO GOOD FOOD, GOOD-BYE PMS!

When it comes to controlling the symptoms of PMS, the importance of a good diet can't be stressed enough. If you eat poorly, there's not a medicine, exercise regime, herb, or alternative technique that can make up for all of the ill effects. Many, many women find that they can either eliminate or markedly reduce their PMS symptoms just by changing their diets. So begin your quest right here, right now, by planning a week's worth of healthy menus for yourself. (It's great eating for your family, too.) Then give it a try. You've got nothing to lose but PMS!

2

Can the Caffeine!

That high-voltage cup of coffee that gets you going in the morning or that great afternoon "pick-me-up" in the form of a can of cola may be doing plenty to exacerbate your PMS, especially if you're a bit of a "caffeine junkie." A study of over two hundred college women found severe PMS symptoms in 60 percent of those who had a daily intake of more than four and one-half cups of caffeine-containing beverages. That's the equivalent of a couple of cups of java with breakfast, a Coke at lunch, and a Mountain Dew at dinner.

WHAT DOES CAFFEINE DO?

Specifically, caffeine can cause irritability, anxiety, mood swings, insomnia, depletion of B vitamins, and breast tenderness. Most of us are familiar with the jangled nerves associated with too much caffeine. But did you know that even small amounts will stimulate the release of the hormone *adrenaline*, the one that gets pumped up when you need to fight or flee? Long used by college students pulling "all-nighter" study sessions, caffeine also helps keep you awake—not necessarily a good thing if you tend to have trouble falling or staying asleep, a common symptom of PMS. It works by increasing production of the neurotransmitter *norepinephrine*, which makes you more alert but can also make you more irritable and anxious. And, since caffeine is metabolized slowly, even drinking one cup of coffee or a soft drink with dinner might keep you from falling asleep at 11:00 P.M.

A natural diuretic, caffeine stimulates the excretion of water, as well as some important vitamins and minerals. B vitamins, magnesium, potassium, zinc, and vitamin C get washed away in the process, and deficiencies of these nutrients are believed to contribute to PMS. B vitamins, for example, are important to glucose metabolism. With a deficiency of these vitamins, you can expect to see blood sugar that soars and crashes, leaving you hungry, shaky, dizzy, etc. The B vitamins are also important for proper function of the liver, which metabolizes estrogen. Without enough B vitamins, estrogen levels can rise too high, leading to water retention, breast tenderness, mood changes, migraine headaches, and sleeplessness. Tender, swollen breasts, in particular, seem to be linked to caffeine intake, with nearly one out of three women finding relief once she cuts caffeine out of her diet.

CAFFEINE HITS HARDER DURING PMS

It's important to remember that it takes longer for your body to break down caffeine during the last two weeks of your menstrual cycle, Days Fourteen to Twenty-Eight (coincidentally the days you're most likely to be affected by PMS). So even if you can get away with caffeine ingestion during the first half of the month, you're more likely to have trouble during the last half. It's best to completely eliminate caffeine from your diet forever, but if you can't do that, at least cut back on your consumption during the two weeks prior to your period.

HOW WE GET OUR CAFFEINE

For most of us, the primary sources of caffeine are the things we drink; namely coffee, tea, and soft drinks. So caffeine intake can usually be cut way back just by switching to decaffeinated beverages. But chocolate, cocoa, and related products also have caffeine, so that cup of hot chocolate before bedtime is probably doing you more harm than good. And don't forget many over-the-counter or prescription medications. Pain relievers (particularly headache remedies) often pack a hefty caffeine punch because it helps constrict painfully throbbing blood vessels.

Caffeine-Containing Foods, Drinks, and Medications	
	Caffeine Content (mg)
Coffee (5 oz. cup)	
Drip	146
Percolated	110
Instant	65
Decaffeinated	3
Tea (5 oz. cup)	
Black (1 min. brew)	28
Black (3 min. brew)	42
Black (5 min. brew)	46
Green (1 min. brew)	14
Green (3 min. brew)	27
Green (5 min. brew)	31
Soft Drinks (12 oz. can)	
Mountain Dew	54
Coca Cola	45
Diet Coke	45
Dr Pepper	42
Pepsi-Cola	38

Caffeine-Containing Foods, Drinks, and Medications *(continued)*	
	Caffeine Content (mg)
Soft Drinks (12 oz. can)	
Diet Pepsi	36
Sprite, 7-Up	0
Cocoa/Chocolate	
Baking chocolate	35
Milk chocolate	6
Sweet, Dark Chocolate	20
Cocoa, dry powder (1 T.)	11
Cocoa beverage (6 oz.)	5
Chocolate cake (1/16 of 9″ cake)	14
Medications	
(Caffeine content listed is for standard dose, unless otherwise noted.)	
NoDoz (stimulant)	200
Vivarin (stimulant)	200
Aqua-Ban (diuretic)	200
Cafergot (migraines, per tablet)	100
Caffedrine (stimulant, per capsule)	200
Dexatrim (weight control)	200
Prolamine (weight control)	200
Excedrin (headaches)	130
Vanquish (headaches)	66
Midol (menstrual pain)	64
Anacin (headaches)	64
Fiorinal (headaches)	40
Esgic (analgesic, per tablet)	40
Darvon (pain, per tablet)	32
Triaminicin (colds)	30

CUTTING BACK ON CAFFEINE

There are loads of brands of decaffeinated coffee, tea, and soft drinks on the market. Decaffeinated coffee is available in just about any restaurant, as is herb tea. (But watch out for mint tea, which does contain caffeine.) You may want to try a grain-based coffee substitute (available in health food stores), such as Postum or Caffix. If you're looking for a stimulant without the caffeine, how about ginger tea? It tastes great and aids digestion at the same time. Best of all, of course, is to substitute plain, delicious water for any of those caffeine-containing drinks. Water washes away toxins and impurities, restores fluid balance, eases constipation, aids in digestion and absorption of food, and is the medium in which the majority of the body's chemical reactions take place. Most of us don't drink enough water, so how about using your caffeine cut-back as an opportunity to increase your water intake?

Just a word of warning, however, before you cut off your caffeine supply completely: if you're used to drinking more than two cups of coffee or a couple of caffeine-containing soft drinks per day, or if you've been taking medications that contain caffeine, don't stop cold turkey! Caffeine is a vasoconstrictor, which means that it narrows your blood vessels. If you're accustomed to the effects of caffeine and you suddenly stop, your blood vessels will widen unnaturally, setting the stage for major headaches. Cut back gradually instead, by substituting a glass or two of water for just *one* of your caffeine-containing beverages. After a week or so, cut out another beverage, and so on.

Don't feel bad if you can't get to the point of being "caffeine-free." Just cutting back on your usual intake can make a positive difference. Aim for a daily intake of 200 mg or less to start with, and see how it goes. (That includes beverages, foods, and medications.) You may find that breast tenderness and anxiety are no longer problems at that level. But if you're still bothered by these symptoms, cut back further over time.

3

Abstain from Alcohol

At first, it might sound like a pretty good idea. You've got PMS, you're irritable, you've just had a fight with your mother over the phone, you feel lousy—hey, how about a glass of wine to mellow out? Well, think again.

WHAT'S WRONG WITH ALCOHOL?

Drinking alcohol can make your PMS symptoms even worse, and it can do so in a variety of ways:

• **Alcohol exacerbates estrogen excess**—Alcohol is a major toxin that must be processed by the liver. But when the liver is overwhelmed by a toxic load, it tends to do a poor job of metabolizing estrogen, allowing excessive levels to build up.

• **Alcohol interferes with absorption and utilization of B vitamins**—The B vitamins play vital roles in the stabilization of blood glucose, the deactivation of estrogen in the liver, and proper function of the neurotransmitters in the brain. If you're low in B vitamins, you're quite likely to be tired, irritable, bloated, and sleepless.

• **Alcohol is destructive to magnesium**—About 80 percent of alcoholics have very low levels of magnesium, and low levels of this mineral have been linked to PMS. Too little magnesium results in decreased levels of dopamine, a neurotransmitter that helps eliminate excess fluid, regulate appetite, and increase mental alertness. Magnesium can also help regulate glucose metabolism, stabilize the mood, and decrease cramps. Without enough magnesium, you can find yourself suffering from mood swings, appetite disturbances, nausea, vomiting, confusion, depression, cramps, loss of coordination, and other unpleasant symptoms.

• **Alcohol interferes with normal glucose metabolism**—Alcohol can cause low blood sugar by blocking the body's normal mechanisms for supplying glucose when it's needed. Or it may throw your blood sugar into a tizzy by driving glucose levels up initially, only to let them crash soon afterward. This is particularly true if you drink forms of alcohol that contain sugar or are mixed with sugary substances. Drinking on an empty stomach will both speed up and increase these effects, leaving you with all the classic signs of hypoglycemia: fatigue, weakness, irritability, and increased aggression. The PMS-related anger experienced by many women who drink alcohol is probably due, in part, to low blood sugar levels. And the "cocktail hour," which often delays mealtime, may further complicate the problem.

• **Alcohol decreases the desire to eat**—After a couple of drinks, a lot of people don't feel like eating. They may pick at their food or skip meals altogether. Those who regularly imbibe often end up substituting alcohol for food, compromising their nutritional status. To make matters worse, many of the nutrients from the foods that they do eat may be malabsorbed, inefficiently used, or lost through urine, vomiting, etc. Yet alcohol itself supplies zero nutrients. Its only nutritional contribution is calories, thus the vitamin and mineral deficiencies so often seen in heavy drinkers.

• **Alcohol is a depressant**—If depression isn't one of your PMS woes, drinking alcohol is a good way to bring it on. The premenstrual phase is a prime time for alcoholism to begin or worsen. Many women start drinking to ease anxiety and tension or to escape from problems. Unfortunately, the resulting depression can become one of their biggest problems since alcohol is a central nervous system depressant and can intensify feelings of hopelessness and despair.

• **Alcohol packs a mightier punch during the PMS phase—** During the week or so before the menstrual period begins, a woman's tolerance to alcohol drops and she may find herself drunk or high on half the number of drinks that it usually takes. Many women find that they cannot control their drinking at this time, although they can at other times of the month.

ADIEU TO ALCOHOL

The best strategy is to try to stay away from alcoholic beverages completely. But if you do want to drink, do so as an *occasional* treat and keep it to one. Sip your drink slowly and sparingly, drink only with a meal and don't drink during your premenstrual phase. The best choices include light beer or light wine as they have less alcohol than the regular varieties. The rest of the time, stick to non-alcoholic choices like sparkling mineral water with a slice of lime, "near beer" (alcohol-free beer), or decaffeinated diet soft drinks.

4

Skip the Sugar

PMS is a complex disorder, with wide-ranging symptoms, causes, and treatments. And while there are still plenty of unsolved mysteries surrounding this condition, medical researchers all seem to agree about one thing: eating sugar makes PMS worse. How unfair that this is exactly the time of the month that you really start craving sweets! I remember buying a box of tampons and a candy bar one time, and the clerk (a woman I knew) remarked wryly, "They should just glue a candy bar on every box of these things, since every woman who buys them also buys something sweet."

THE SWEET TOOTH PROBLEM

As mentioned in Chapter 1, during the week before your period, your body becomes extra responsive to insulin, the hormone that clears glucose from your blood and sends it into the cells, where it's used for energy. But the insulin can clear away too much glucose, leaving you with unnaturally low blood sugar, a condition called *hypoglycemia*. Suddenly, you feel tired, shaky, hungry, irritable, and moody. Your brain signals the body that it needs more fuel, and you begin to crave sweets. This is also the time when many women crave chocolate, and with good reason. Besides being high in sugar, chocolate contains magnesium (a mineral that's often deficient during the premenstrual phase) and *phenylethylamine*, an amino acid that helps ease depression. No wonder women like chocolate so much! But, alas, eating chocolate or any other high-sugar food is the last thing you need when you're premenstrual and dying for something sweet. That's because:

• **Sugar makes you moody, irritable, fatigued, and weak**—Eating sugar stimulates the release of large amounts of insulin, the same substance that's causing your blood sugar to plummet in the first place. So what do you do as your blood sugar takes yet another nosedive? You eat more sugar! It's a vicious circle that can keep you feeling edgy throughout the entire PMS phase.

• **Sugar can exacerbate estrogen excess**—Too much sugar overworks the liver, making it less able to process estrogen effectively. Estrogen levels rise, and you end up feeling bloated, irritable, and anxious.

• **Sugar increases feelings of anxiety**—The blood glucose crash that follows an overload of sugar activates your adrenal glands, which release adrenaline to push your blood glucose back up. But adrenaline increases anxiety and stimulates the release of another hormone, *cortisol*, which causes intense cravings for—what else?—sugar.

• **Sugar can worsen progesterone deficiency**—Besides increasing anxiety, a rise in cortisol has the undesirable side effect of lowering progesterone and raising estrogen. Cortisol also makes it harder for your body to use progesterone efficiently. So even if your body manages to make adequate levels of progesterone, at least some of it can't be used properly.

• **Sugar works against good nutrition**—Excessive amounts of sugar can deplete the body of B vitamins, chromium, magnesium, zinc, and copper. And sugary foods tend to replace nutritious foods in the diet, leading to a greater chance of deficiencies that, in turn, can bring on the symptoms of PMS and other conditions.

The solution: avoid sugar and sugary substances like the plague, especially during the week or so before your period. Instead, when you feel your blood sugar slipping, eat something containing complex carbohydrates, like whole-grain breads, cereal or pasta, beans, peas, and other legumes. Remember that fruits and, to a lesser extent, vegetables contain natural sugars that can drive up blood glucose levels. So always eat fruits or vegetables in conjunction with a small amount of protein (cottage cheese is a good protein source) and/or some complex carbohydrate, both of which will slow the entrance of glucose into the bloodstream.

SUGAR-CONTAINING FOODS AND DRINKS

Do your best to limit or avoid the following high-sugar foods:

- Breakfast cereals (most of them)
- Cakes
- Candy
- Catsup
- Chewing gum (sweetened)
- Cookies
- Desserts
- Fruit canned in syrup
- Fruit punch
- Gelatin desserts
- Honey
- Ice cream
- Jams
- Jellies
- Preserves
- Pudding
- Relish

- Salad dressing
- Soft drinks (non-diet kind)
- Syrups
- Table sugar
- Yogurt (sweetened)

NOTE: Refined foods like white bread, white rice, instant potatoes, or cornflakes can act like sugar in the system because of their lack of fiber. Your blood sugar can soar after eating these foods by themselves, as if you'd eaten a candy bar. It's best to stick to whole-grain foods, since their high fiber content allows them to enter the bloodstream more slowly. If you do eat refined foods like the ones listed above, eat some high-protein, high-fiber foods at the same time to keep your blood sugar from skyrocketing.

HELP WITH LOWERING YOUR SUGAR INTAKE

If you want to get a handle on your intake of sugar, the first thing you need to do is become an avid label-reader. Sugar hides in practically all processed foods, and you just might not recognize it in its current "incarnation." When you're reading the food label on a package or a can, don't think that a food is sugar-free just because the word "sugar" isn't listed. Sugar has many different names, including the following:

By Any Other Name, It's Still . . . Sugar!
- Brown sugar
- Concentrated fruit juice
- Corn syrup
- Dextrose
- Fructose
- Glucose
- High fructose corn syrup
- Honey

- Lactose
- Maltodextrin
- Maltose
- Molasses
- Raw sugar
- Sucrose

Whenever you see any of the above as one of the first four ingredients on the label (meaning it's one of the main ingredients), put it back on the shelf—it's definitely a high-sugar food.

You can also help lower your sugar intake by making a few easy changes. Begin by getting rid of your sugar bowl so you won't be tempted to add sugar to your food at the table. Always opt for fresh fruit rather than canned, but if you do buy canned, get the kind that's packed in water or fruit juice rather than syrup. Try the low-sugar versions of jams and jellies—many are quite tasty. And for snacking, plain popcorn or unsalted nuts are much better choices than candy.

While you should limit your consumption of baked goods and desserts, when you do want something sweet, how about plain angel food cake with fresh fruit instead of a piece of frosted layer cake? And if you just can't live without cookies, at least avoid chocolate chip, sandwich style, or the chocolate-covered kind, substituting plain graham crackers, vanilla wafers, or gingersnaps.

You can do plenty to reduce the sugar content of the foods you prepare at home. Cinnamon, cardamom, ginger, nutmeg, and other spices give a "sweet" flavor without adding sugar. Try using small amounts of these spices to replace some of the sugar in certain recipes. In general, you can probably cut back on the amount of sugar you use in cooking without significantly affecting the taste. Try it! Reduce the sugar in your favorite recipe by one-fourth at first and decide if the taste is still acceptable. If so, reduce a little more next time until you figure out how far you can go without ruining the recipe. You may be surprised at how much unnecessary sugar your recipes contain!

You may think I'm crazy for suggesting that you cut back on sugar at the exact time of the month that you're dying for it! But your cravings should actually recede once you stop eating a lot of refined sugar, especially if you're eating six wholesome, nutritious, and balanced meals each day, as suggested in Chapter 1. The sad truth is that sugar is not your friend. It's your enemy, especially during the PMS phase of your cycle.

5

Shun the Salt

If you've got problems with premenstrual water retention, bloating, weight gain, breast swelling and/or breast tenderness, remember: wherever salt goes, water follows. But, then, you already know this. Whenever you're eating something salty, say potato chips or pretzels, what's the first thing you reach for? A soft drink, a beer, or a big glass of water. That's because your body needs to keep its water-to-sodium ratio in balance in order to function properly. So the input of extra sodium naturally triggers the input of extra water.

The same thing happens inside your tissues. The greater the density of sodium, the greater the amount of water pulled into your tissues to balance it. So if you tend to retain water, the more sodium you consume, the worse your problem will get—or so the theory goes. Nobody's actually proved this, but it certainly makes sense.

HOW MUCH IS TOO MUCH?

The average person needs to take in only about 500 mg of sodium per day (the equivalent of about ¼ tsp. of salt) to maintain health.

But according to recent estimates, most people take in as much as ten to twenty times that amount—somewhere in the range of 5 to 10 grams per day! The U.S. Dietary Guideline Committee recommends limiting sodium intake to six grams or less as a guideline for general health, since high levels of sodium are associated with high blood pressure, kidney disease, and liver disease.

For those who have water retention problems, six grams of sodium (6,000 mg) per day is probably still too much—4 grams (4,000 mg) or less is a better idea. But it will take more than just staying away from the salt shaker to cut your sodium down to that level. Sodium lurks in practically everything we eat, even fresh fruits and vegetables. Still, no one's suggesting you give up sodium completely. Just be aware of which foods have high, moderate, and low sodium contents and try to emphasize those that are moderate to low, while avoiding or restricting those that are high.

To give you an idea of how salt and salty substances translate into milligrams of sodium, consider the following:

Food Item	Sodium (in mg)
1 tsp. of salt	2,000
1 tsp. baking soda	1,000
4 oz. baked ham	1,027
1 dill pickle	928
1 cup vegetable soup	838
2 oz. corned beef	535
8 oz. buttermilk	319
2 slices white bread	292
1 baking powder biscuit	272
½ cup tomato juice	243

Take a look at the following table to see which common foods are classified as high-, moderate-, and low-sodium.

High-Sodium Foods (more than 400 mg sodium per serving)	Moderate-Sodium Foods (between 100 and 400 mg sodium per serving)	Low-Sodium Foods (less than 100 mg per serving)
Baking soda	Baking powder	Beverages, carbonated
Canned meats and/or fish	Beet greens	Bread and crackers, low sodium
Cereal, instant	Biscuits, muffins	Butter or margarine, unsalted
Cheese (American, bleu, Roquefort, cottage, parmesan)	Bread, rolls	Cereals: hot (except instant), puffed wheat or rice, shredded wheat
Crackers and chips, salted	Butter or margarine, salted	Cheese: Gruyere, ricotta, Swiss, unsalted, cream cheese
Frozen dinners	Buttermilk	Cream
Meats (smoked, cured, or pickled)	Cakes, pies, pastries	Eggs
Pasta dishes, commercially prepared	Catsup	Flour
Pickled vegetables, olives, sauerkraut	Celery	Fruit juice
Popcorn, salted	Cereal, dry	Fruit, fresh
Pretzels, salted	Chard	Grains, unsalted
Salt	Cheese (except Swiss, ricotta, Gruyere and cream cheese)	Matzah
Salty seasonings (bouillon, garlic salt, onion salt, soy sauce, teriyaki sauce)	Chili sauce	Meats, fish and poultry, fresh (prepared without salt)
Soup, packaged or canned	Custard	Pasta
Vegetable juice, salted	Gravy	Peanut butter, unsalted
	Ice cream	Peas and beans, dried
	Mayonnaise	Popcorn, unsalted
	Milk (all kinds)	Seasonings, unsalted (i.e., basil, cinnamon, cloves, dill, pepper, paprika, garlic, etc.)
	Monosodium glutamate (MSG)	Tortillas, corn
	Mustard	Vegetable juice, unsalted
	Nuts and seeds, salted	Vegetables, fresh (except celery, beet greens, chard)
	Pancakes, waffles	
	Peanut butter, salted	
	Peas, frozen	
	Pudding	
	Salad dressings, commercial	
	Shellfish, fresh	
	Soy sauce, low sodium	
	Vegetables, canned	
	Worcestershire sauce	
	Yogurt	

THE RULES

The truth of the matter is, eating a truly "low-sodium" diet is about the hardest thing in the world. Food tastes really bland without any added sodium, so I don't advise that you restrict yourself too severely. Instead, begin by following these simple rules:

Dos
- Do use salt in cooking and baking, but try to cut the amount down by half.
- Do substitute the following seasonings for salt to flavor your food whenever possible: allspice, basil, bay leaf, chives, cinnamon, dill, garlic powder, lemon juice, marjoram, mint, nutmeg, onion powder, oregano, paprika, parsley, rosemary, sage, or thyme.
- Do limit your intake of baking soda and baking powder.

Don'ts
- Don't add salt to your food at the table. (Throw away your salt shaker!)
- Don't use canned broth or soup unless it's the low-sodium kind.
- Don't eat foods that have been preserved with salt, such as bacon, bologna, ham, and sausage.
- Don't eat salty foods like potato chips, salted crackers, or salted nuts.
- Don't eat pickled foods like pickles, olives, pickled vegetables, pickled herring, or sauerkraut.
- Don't use salty seasonings like garlic salt, onion salt, seasoned salt, meat tenderizer, MSG, soy sauce, teriyaki sauce, or bouillon.

"LIMIT" DOESN'T MEAN "ELIMINATE"

Begin your quest for lower sodium intake by sticking to these rules and choosing your diet from the moderate- to low-sodium foods listed above. But if you find yourself feeling so deprived that you're tempted to forget the whole thing, go ahead and relax the rules a bit until you feel more comfortable. The idea is to *decrease* the amount of sodium that you normally consume, not to win the title for consuming the world's lowest-sodium diet! A gradual downward trend is the goal.

Follow your new lower-sodium plan for at least a month and see if it helps ease your water-retention problem. If it doesn't, consider cutting back a bit more. Then, if you still don't see or feel any results, your problem may not be due to excessive salt intake. But don't go back to your old high-sodium ways. Experts agree that for general health purposes a moderate intake of sodium is best.

6

Eat More Fiber

My grandmother used to call it "roughage," others have called it "bulk," and many people think it's synonymous with bran cereal. Whichever way you say it or see it, fiber is a catchall term that refers to the indigestible parts of plants. Some of these plant parts act like little brooms that sweep through the digestive system, clearing out wastes and toxins and speeding up the transit time of food as it passes through the intestines. Others act like little sponges, soaking up bile acids, cholesterol, and deactivated estrogen, which are then excreted rather than reabsorbed. So eating good amounts of fiber can play some important roles in preventing several serious diseases, including cancer, diabetes, and heart disease.

There are two main types of fiber: *insoluble* (meaning it won't dissolve in water) and *soluble* (meaning it will). The insoluble kind is chewy and coarse, and is found in wheat bran, leafy green vegetables, and the skins of fruits and root vegetables. It bulks up the stool, absorbs water, and stimulates contraction of the intestinal walls so wastes are pushed through faster. Intestinal wastes are full of toxins and the longer they are in contact with the walls of the colon, the greater the chance of the development of colon cancer. But a diet high in insoluble fiber speeds the intestinal contents through, and may be the best protection against colon cancer.

Soluble fiber, on the other hand, includes some plant parts that can be dissolved in water such as pectin, gums, and mucilage. The most famous member of this family is oat bran, a cereal that got movie-star billing in the 1980s as a fast and easy way to lower blood cholesterol. Sources of soluble fiber include oats, beans, barley, psyllium seed, and many vegetables and fruits.

WHAT DOES FIBER DO TO HELP EASE PMS?

While just about everybody knows that fiber is good for bulking up the stool and preventing constipation, many people are unaware that it can also do plenty to lessen the symptoms of PMS.

• **Fiber helps decrease excess estrogen**—A high-fiber diet can help counteract one of the most likely causes of PMS—estrogen excess. It works like this: once estrogen completes its duties, it goes to the liver to become deactivated, then is excreted through the digestive system. But a high-fat diet can *re*activate estrogen in the intestinal tract and send it right back into the bloodstream, driving up the levels of circulating estrogen and bringing on symptoms of PMS. The more time that digestive wastes spend sitting in your colon, the greater the re-absorption of this "old estrogen." But if you eat foods containing soluble fiber, it will bind to estrogen in the intestinal tract and sweep it out of the body along with other digestive wastes.

• **A high-fiber diet helps improve glucose tolerance**—Soluble fiber, when combined with water, forms a gel-like substance in the intestines that slows the rate of digestion. That means that glucose is released into your bloodstream more slowly. Since many women have trouble with fluctuating blood glucose levels during the PMS phase, this is a real plus. Fiber also helps keep glucose levels stable by altering certain hormones in the gut, which improve glucose metabolism in the liver. The upshot of all this is you'll have fewer mood swings, more energy, and less desire to binge on sweets.

• **Fiber reduces the urge to binge by adding bulk to the food mix, which gives a feeling of fullness**—Think about how full you'd feel after eating three slices of whole wheat bread. Now imagine how full you'd feel after eating a candy bar, which contains roughly the same amount of calories, but a lot less fiber. A high-fiber diet fills you up and takes time to consume. If you're eating six to eleven servings of whole grains and at least five servings of fruits and vegetables every day, you're probably not going to be inclined to top it off with a box of cookies or half of a chocolate cake! So on a high-fiber diet, you'll probably find yourself eating more food but taking in fewer calories.

• **Fiber helps the body fully utilize progesterone**—Some experts theorize that the highs and lows in blood sugar experienced by many women during the PMS phase result in a release of adrenaline to boost blood sugar levels. Unfortunately, extra adrenaline makes it hard for the body to use progesterone in an efficient way—which amounts to the same thing as progesterone deficiency. But by eating a high-fiber diet, blood sugar levels are stabilized and hormone levels follow suit.

HOW MUCH FIBER IS ENOUGH?

The average American consumes about eleven grams of fiber a day, an amount that experts consider shockingly low. Most authorities recommend at least double that amount, if not more—between twenty and thirty grams per day. Some push for even higher amounts, but forty-five grams seems to be the upper limit. Too much fiber can result in intestinal gas and irritation, bloating, diarrhea, impaction of the feces, and even a ruptured bowel, so don't go overboard. It's best to increase your fiber intake gradually; don't start eating thirty grams of fiber tomorrow if you're used to taking in only eleven grams. And be sure to drink at least eight glasses of water per day. Fiber draws water, so you'll need to drink up in order to process it properly.

Some Good Sources of Fiber		
Moderate Amounts (3.1–4.0 grams fiber)	**Moderately High Amounts** (4.1–6.0 grams fiber)	**High Amounts** (6.1 or more grams fiber)
Beets, ½ c.	Beet greens, ½ c.	All-Bran cereal, ½ c
Bread, whole-wheat, 1 slice	Beans, lentils (cooked) ½ c.	Artichoke, 1
Bread, rye, 1 slice	Broccoli, ¾ c.	Berries, ½ c.
Cashews, 6–8	Green beans, ½ c.	Currants, dried, ¼ c.
Cereal, rolled oats, ¾ c. cooked	Nuts (most kinds) 2 oz.	Legumes (garbanzo beans,
Cereal, 40% bran, 1 c.	Potato, sweet, 1 sm.	lima beans,
Orange, 1 med.	Parsnip, 1 large	soybeans) ½ c.
Potato, white, 1 med. w/skin	Prunes, 6	Bran muffin, 1
		Pumpkin, ½ c.
		Sunflower seeds, 1 oz.

ADDING FIBER TO YOUR DIET

Adopting the diet outlined in Chapter 1 is a good place to start if you want to increase your fiber intake. But even when you faithfully eat six to eleven servings of grains and at least five fruits and vegetables per day, if your grains are primarily the refined kind (white flour, white rice, instant cereal, etc.) and your fruits and vegetables are canned or otherwise processed, you may not be getting enough fiber. When you're thinking about adding fiber to your diet, it's important to remember two things:

• **Fiber comes from plant products, not animal products**—You won't find dietary fiber in any significant amount in meats, fish, poultry, dairy products, eggs, cheese, or any other animal product unless it's mixed with plant products. So even though beef jerky may *seem* fibrous, it's devoid of dietary fiber.

• **The closer the plant product comes to being in its natural, unprocessed form, the more fiber it will have**—Soybeans have a lot more fiber than textured soy protein. Raw carrots have more fiber than cooked carrots. If you can eat your fruits and vegetables raw, do so. (Obviously, you can't eat potatoes or dried beans raw, so don't try.) But make allowances for taste, too. If you enjoy raw vegetables, then munch away. But if they're unappealing to you, feel free to cook them. The idea is to get you to eat plentiful amounts of nutritious foods— but you're not going to do that if you find them unpalatable.

While keeping these two things in mind, try to include a wide variety of fiber-rich foods in your diet. That way, you'll get both soluble and insoluble fiber, plus a mix of other nutrients. Always opt for whole grains rather than refined grains whenever possible, and read the labels on your bread, cereals, rice, pasta, and crackers. (If the first ingredient isn't a whole grain, find another brand!) Eat a hot or cold bran cereal at breakfast, since bran cereals offer more fiber than just about anything else, and eat the skin on fruits and vegetables whenever possible. Foods should be consumed in their least-processed state (an apple has a lot more fiber than apple juice), so go for the whole food whenever you can and try to distribute fiber-rich foods throughout the day. It's way too much to consume twenty grams of fiber at breakfast and next to nothing during the rest of the day. Your digestive system will thank you if you eat small amounts of fiber several times a day. Finally, drink plenty of water or other liquids. Eating a lot of fiber without enough liquid can lead to serious digestive problems.

It's possible to get fiber from bulk laxatives (psyllium seed is often a major ingredient) or from pills, but you won't get the nutrients or the satisfied feeling you'd get from eating fiber-rich foods. Real food is always your best bet.

7

Eat the "Good" Fats

If you're like me, you've probably spent your adult life trying to avoid fat, the great enemy of weight watchers and health seekers the world over. "Fat makes you fat," so the saying goes, not to mention the role it plays in clogging arteries and bringing on heart disease and certain types of cancer. But in recent years, researchers have determined that all fats are *not* created equal. There are, in fact, certain fats that can be considered "good," especially if you suffer from PMS. That's because many PMS sufferers have a fatty-acid profile that's out of whack—that is, the amounts and kinds of fatty acids flowing through their bloodstreams are different from those found in other people.

TOO LITTLE GLA CAN TRIGGER PMS

Specifically, researchers found that women with PMS have exceedingly low levels of a fatty acid called *gamma-linoleic acid* (GLA), to the point where their GLA levels may be barely detectable! Why is this important? If your GLA levels are too low, your body starts to produce excessive amounts of *prolactin*, the hormone known best for "turning on" milk production in the breasts after a baby has been delivered. These high levels of prolactin interfere with the production of progesterone, causing an imbalance between your estrogen and progesterone levels. That translates to the symptoms of estrogen dominance and PMS: water retention, weight gain, tissue swelling, breast tenderness, anxiety, fatigue, low blood sugar, and all the rest.

As if that weren't enough, low GLA levels contribute to pain and inflammation through their role in the production of hormone-like substances called *prostaglandins*. There are two main types of prostaglandins, PG-1 and PG-2. Both regulate several vital processes, and the two tend to work in opposition. You can think of PG-1 as the "inflammation fighting" prostaglandin, while PG-2 is the "inflammation producing" kind. So while PG-1 helps decrease inflammation, relax the uterus, improve blood flow, reduce cramping, and ease swelling and breast tenderness, PG-2 has just the opposite effect, increasing inflammation and bloating, stimulating uterine contractions, and slowing the flow of blood. PG-2 also increases your body's production of both cortisol (the stress hormone) and estrogen, each of which contributes to progesterone deficiency. So if you've either got too little of PG-1 or too much of PG-2, you can find yourself in PMS hell!

FORTIFYING YOUR GLA SUPPLY

Since GLA helps increase your supply of the "good" prostaglandins, it makes sense to ensure that you get plentiful amounts of this fatty acid. Excellent sources of GLA include evening primrose oil, black currant oil, and borage seed oil. Many women have enjoyed relief from their PMS symptoms (especially breast tenderness) just by taking a dose of one of these oils during the premenstrual phase. In a study done in 1982, sixty-eight women with PMS took one to two grams of evening primrose oil, beginning three days prior to the time that PMS symptoms usually appeared and continuing until their menstrual periods began. After three months of treatment, complete relief of PMS symptoms was reported by 61 percent of the women, and 23 percent reported partial relief. Breast tenderness was the symptom that was relieved most dramatically. While not all studies of evening primrose oil have shown such positive results, it does seem to be safe when taken at a dose of between two and four grams daily.

You may be able to get similar results by increasing your intake of linoleic acid, the stuff your body uses to manufacture GLA. Some experts estimate that up to 80 percent of us aren't getting enough linoleic acid, thus our society's widespread deficiency in GLA and our lack of "good" prostaglandins. You can get plenty of linoleic acid by including one tablespoon of light vegetable oils like safflower, corn, sunflower, or soy oil in your daily diet.

But the simplest solution of all may be to take flaxseed oil, which not only contains plenty of linoleic acid but is also an excellent source of omega-3 fatty acids. (See section below.) And it's a lot less expensive than evening primrose, black currant, or borage seed oils.

FISHING FOR RELIEF

If you suspect that an overload of PG-2 (inflammatory prostaglandins) might be the cause of your PMS, you may also want to include the "big gun" of dietary anti-inflammatories in your diet: omega-3 fatty acids. Not only do the omega-3s decrease inflammation, they can help stabilize blood sugar, fight premenstrual acne, increase production of endorphins (the "feel-good hormones"), and improve the action of other hormones. Omega-3 fatty acids can be found in the fat or oil of cold water fish such as anchovies, herring, mackerel, rockfish, salmon, sardines, tuna, and whitefish. Studies of fish oil supplements show that they can ease the symptoms of several inflammation-related conditions, including rheumatoid arthritis, migraine headaches, and PMS. (Conversely, in one study of Danish women, those with *lower* dietary levels of omega-3 fatty acids were found to have *more* menstrual pain.) And fish oil is an excellent source of vitamin D, which helps the body absorb calcium and magnesium.

To make sure you're getting enough omega-3 fatty acids, eat two to five (cold water) fish meals per week (but don't fry the fish; it destroys the omega-3s). Other good sources include black walnuts, butter nuts, and green soybeans. Surprisingly, the most potent version of the omega-3s is *not* fish or fish oil, but our old friend, flaxseed oil, which contains more than twice as many omega-3s. So by taking flaxseed oil, you'll get a 2-for-1 bonus: a rich source of omega 3s that can also provide your body with the building blocks of GLA. Generally, either eating plenty of fish, taking fish oil, or taking flaxseed oil will provide you with a sufficient amount of omega-3 fatty acids.

WARNING: Both fish oil and GLA supplements thin the blood, and large doses of either can result in uncontrolled bleeding. If you're taking blood-thinning medications, non-steroidal anti-inflammatory medications, supplements that contain ginger, or anything else that thins the blood, consult your doctor before taking fish oil or GLA. Do not take a full dose of both kinds of supplements at the same time. Take one or the other or take half-doses of each.

WATCH YOUR SATURATED FAT INTAKE

The other thing you need to remember when increasing your "good" prostaglandins while decreasing the "bad," is to watch your intake of saturated fat (the kind found in red meat, cheese, bacon, lard, or full-fat dairy products.) This also holds true for hydrogenated fat (the kind found in margarine or shortening) and rancid vegetable oils. All of these fats can contribute to the overproduction of PG-2, the "inflammation-producing" kind of prostaglandin, so forgo the bacon cheeseburger in favor of some nice broiled fish.

ALL YOU REALLY NEED TO KNOW . . .

If all of this sounds like too much scientific mumbo-jumbo, here's a summary of the most important parts:

- PMS sufferers appear to have abnormal levels of certain fats in the blood.
- These abnormal fat levels can cause estrogen dominance and/or progesterone deficiency, both of which bring on PMS symptoms.
- You can help normalize your blood fats and balance your hormones by:
  1. Taking 1 T. of flaxseed oil (or 1,000 mg in capsule form) daily *or* a GLA supplement (evening primrose oil, borage seed oil, or black currant oil) *or* increasing your intake of linoleic acid (light oils like safflower, sunflower, or soy oil)
  2. Avoiding saturated fat.
- Omega-3 fatty acids can help ease inflammation, regulate your blood sugar, improve hormonal function, fight premenstrual acne, and increase endorphin levels. You can get plenty of omega-3 fatty acids by:
  1. Eating two to five fish meals per week, especially cold water fish like anchovies, herring, salmon, mackerel, tuna, etc.
  2. Eating black walnuts, green soybeans, butter nuts, or other plant sources of omega-3 fatty acids.
  3. Taking one T. of fish oil or the equivalent of fish oil supplements, if you're *not* already taking flaxseed oil or eating plenty of fish.

Remember, fat can be a good thing if it's the right kind of fat, taken in the right amount. But either too much or too little can upset your body's delicate balance and bring on PMS symptoms or make them worse.

8

Phytoestrogens

Phytoestrogens are literally "plant estrogens," substances found in certain plants that exert an estrogen-like effect on the body. While not chemically identical to estrogen, they can function like the hormone inside our bodies.

To understand how this works, you need to know a little bit about the way hormones function. To begin with, the estrogen that's manufactured inside your body doesn't just flow in and out of the body's cells at will. The cell has to "decide" that's it's okay to let the estrogen in. But first, the estrogen must prove that it belongs there.

You can think of a molecule of estrogen as a little key that floats through the bloodstream in search of a particular kind of lock. A cell that uses estrogen will have that special kind of "lock," called an *estrogen receptor site*. The estrogen "key" floats along, discovers the special "lock," and inserts itself. Voila! The cell is "unlocked," allowing the estrogen to enter. Like an exclusive nightclub, the cell ensures that only the "proper clientele" can enter.

A KEY TO ACHIEVING HEALTHY ESTROGEN LEVELS

Phytoestrogens can also be thought of as keys that float through the bloodstream. Although not identical to estrogen, phytoestrogens will fit into the special estrogen receptor site. But the hormonal effect of the phytoestrogens is about four hundred times *less* than that of human estrogen. And, as it turns out, this is good for women who have estrogen levels that are either too low *or* too high.

How could it be good for both? If you have too little estrogen, the phytoestrogens will boost your estrogen levels, helping to alleviate menstrual irregularities, hot flashes, vaginal dryness, depression, irritability, and the like. But if you've got too much estrogen, the phytoestrogen keys will compete with your natural estrogen for receptor site locks. That means that less of your natural estrogen will get into the cells and the phytoestrogens that take its place will exert a much weaker hormonal effect. The result is lower estrogen levels overall. In short, phytoestrogens appear to have the ability to balance your estrogen levels, whether they're high or low. In addition, they may help prevent breast, prostate, and certain other kinds of cancer that are hormonally triggered, while simultaneously lowering elevated triglyceride and cholesterol levels.

TWO KINDS OF PHYTOESTROGENS

The phytoestrogens come in two forms: isoflavones and lignans. Isoflavones are primarily found in soybeans and soy products such as soy milk, soy flour, tofu, miso, tempeh, and natto. Lignans are found in whole grains, flaxseed, and (in lesser amounts) in alfalfa, celery, parsley, apples, and nuts. Phytoestrogens can also be found in certain herbs, such as black cohosh, licorice root, anise, and fennel.

GETTING PHYTOESTROGENS INTO YOUR DIET

Although supplements containing soy isoflavones are currently on the market, some experts advise against them, saying that too many soy chemicals may reduce the body's ability to absorb minerals, contribute to thyroid abnormalities, cause a decline in mental abilities, and even increase the risk of breast cancer and pancreatic cancer. The best way to increase your intake of phytoestrogens is to eat a diet rich in plant foods—vegetables, fruits, and whole grains—and eat a couple of servings of a soy-based food each week.

9

Vitamins

If you're eating the kinds and amounts of foods outlined in Chapter 1, plus plenty of fiber, "good" fats, and phytoestrogens, while simultaneously limiting your sugar, salt, caffeine, and alcohol intake, you might well assume that you don't need any vitamin supplements. But there are two reasons that you should be taking them anyway. First, vitamins can act as a kind of nutritional insurance against the stress, toxins, and environmental insults that slowly nibble away at your good health. Second, researchers theorize that certain vitamin deficiencies may either cause PMS or make it worse. And for those of you who *don't* eat perfectly, vitamin supplements can help supply what's missing in your diet. Just make sure you don't use supplements as an excuse to pass up nutritious foods while heading for the fatty, sugary, or highly refined kind. There's a lot more to food than just vitamin content, and the nutrients that you actually eat are bound to make the biggest impact on your health.

That said, let's focus on the effects of vitamins on PMS. Following is a list of the vitamin supplements that are most useful in treating PMS symptoms, what they do, and their recommended dosages.

VITAMIN A/BETA-CAROTENE

What it does in general: Vitamin A (which comes from animal sources) and its alter ego, beta-carotene (which comes from plant sources and is converted to vitamin A within the body), function as antioxidant, antistress vitamins that help prevent tumor growth; keep skin, eyes, and mucous membranes healthy; and ward off infection. A deficiency of vitamin A has been linked to PMS. While too much Vitamin A can cause serious side effects like liver damage and malformation of the fetus, it's practically impossible to overdose on beta-carotene. The worst side effect of too much beta-carotene is a temporary case of yellowish skin.

How it can ease PMS: Vitamin A helps fight premenstrual acne, while both A and beta-carotene fight free-radical action and support the production of progesterone.

Recommended Dosage for PMS: Vitamin A = 10,000 I.U. and beta-carotene = 15,000 I.U. daily. Women of child-bearing age shouldn't take more than 2,500 I.U. of Vitamin A, in case a pregnancy occurs.

Food sources: Beta-carotene comes from plant sources such as carrots, butternut squash, sweet potatoes, broccoli, and apricots. Vitamin A comes from animal sources such as fish and fish oil, liver, and egg yolk.

VITAMIN B COMPLEX

What it does in general: Vitamin B complex is a group of B vitamins that work together to accomplish several vital tasks in the body, including the metabolism of protein, fats, and carbohydrates. B vitamins also play an important part in the healthy functioning of the liver and adrenal glands and help stabilize brain chemistry. The vitamins in the B-complex group are typically found together in food and include thiamin, riboflavin, niacin, biotin, pantothenic acid, vitamin B$_6$, PABA, choline, inositol, vitamin B$_{12}$, and folic acid.

How it can ease PMS: Because it aids in the metabolism of carbohydrates, B complex can help stabilize blood sugar, ease mood swings, decrease sugar cravings, improve sleep, and fight fatigue and insomnia. It also helps the liver deactivate and dispose of old estrogen, which helps guard against estrogen buildup. B complex also supports adrenal function, decreasing inflammation, sugar cravings, and headaches.

Recommended Dosage for PMS: Look for a B complex supplement containing 50 mg of most of the major B vitamins—thiamin, riboflavin, niacinamide, pantothenic acid, PABA, choline, and inositol. Take one or two daily.

NOTE: Make sure your niacin is in the form of niacinamide, which can help support production of an important hormone/neurotransmitter called serotonin.

Food sources: Whole grains, liver, brewer's yeast, legumes.

VITAMIN B$_6$

What it does in general: Although B$_6$ is part of the B complex, its role in preventing PMS is so important that it bears a more detailed mention here. In general, B$_6$ is involved in protein and carbohydrate metabolism, the manufacture of neurotransmitters (chemicals in the brain that affect nerve function) and the formation of hemoglobin, among other things.

How it can ease PMS: Some cases of PMS have been associated with a deficiency in B$_6$, which is necessary for production of the neurotransmitters dopamine and serotonin. These two substances are important regulators of mood, memory, water balance, and sleep, and if they're in short supply, you're not going to be feeling very well. Studies have shown that taking 50 mg of B$_6$ throughout the month, then increasing the dosage slightly just before menstruation, can help ease depression, irritability, mood swings, breast tenderness, fatigue, sugar cravings, acne, and water retention. B_6 also plays a part in producing the "good" kind of prostaglandins and helps maintain a healthy estrogen/progesterone balance, which can ease headaches, insomnia, and anxiety.

Recommended Dosage for PMS: 50–200 mg per day. If you're already taking a B complex with 50 mg of B_6, consider adding another 50 mg of B_6 during the premenstrual phase only.

WARNING: Nerve damage occurs when B_6 is taken at doses greater than 500 mg, but some people experience nerve problems at levels as low as 50 mg. Consult with your doctor before taking B_6. If you and your physician decide that you should take this vitamin, gradually add it to your diet and watch for reactions, particularly numbness or tingling in the hands or feet.

Food sources: Salmon, tuna, chicken, soybeans, kale, lentils, whole-wheat flour, brown rice, spinach, broccoli, bananas, sunflower seeds.

VITAMIN C

What it does in general: Vitamin C functions as an antioxidant and an antistress vitamin that helps boost general immune function. It's necessary for the production of collagen (a major ingredient in the body's connective tissue), support of the adrenal glands (especially during times of stress), and the manufacture of certain hormones and neurotransmitters.

How it can ease PMS: Vitamin C aids in adrenal function, thereby fighting fatigue, aches and pains, sugar cravings, and allergies, and boosting the immune system. It can also lessen water retention, ease breast swelling, and assist the liver in breaking down estrogen.

Recommended Dosage for PMS: 500 mg to 3 grams daily.

Food sources: Brussels sprouts, cantaloupe, red pepper, citrus fruits, green pepper, cabbage, kale, raspberries, tomatoes, potatoes, dark green and yellow leafy vegetables.

VITAMIN E

What it does in general: Vitamin E is a potent antioxidant that improves immune function. It also helps protect vitamin A and unsaturated fats from breaking down inside the body. Vitamin E is crucial in the maintenance of healthy tissue in the eyes, skin, breasts, muscles, and liver. Studies have shown that it has a protective effect against cancer and heart disease, it safeguards red blood cells, and it improves the efficiency of insulin.

How it can ease PMS: Vitamin E is of great help in easing breast tenderness. Studies of women who had premenstrual breast tenderness showed that they found substantial relief after two months of taking 300 I.U. of vitamin E daily. It also plays a role in the formation of PG-1 (the beneficial kind of prostaglandin that can ease inflammation and cramps), and may be helpful in relieving depression, insomnia, and fatigue.

Recommended Dosage for PMS: 400–1,600 I.U. daily.

Food sources: Wheat-germ oil, walnut oil, sweet potatoes, safflower oil, turnip greens, beet greens, asparagus, corn oil, broccoli, green leafy vegetables, green beans, nuts, and seeds.

PUTTING IT ALL TOGETHER

It's really not necessary to take sixty-two different vitamin pills in order to get what you need to maintain your health and help ward off certain PMS symptoms. Most of what you need can be found in a high-quality multivitamin. Then add additional supplements as needed. My recommendations for vitamin supplementation are as follows:

Beta-carotene	15,000 I.U.
Vitamin A	2,500–10,000 I.U.
Thiamin	50–100 mg
Riboflavin	50–100 mg
Niacinamide	50–100 mg
Pantothenic acid	50–100 mg
Vitamin B_6	50–200 mg
Choline	50–100 mg
Inositol	50–100 mg
PABA	50–100 mg
Folic acid	400–800 mcg
Biotin	50–100 mcg
Vitamin B_{12}	50–100 mcg
Vitamin C	500–3,000 mg
Vitamin D	400 I.U.
Vitamin E	400–1,000 I.U.

10

Minerals

Minerals are vital to normal cell function and the maintenance of healthy bones, teeth, and body tissues. They also play an important part in protein, fat, and carbohydrate metabolism; hormone production; and the regulation of immune function.

The minerals work together in a balanced, cooperative way, like members of a symphony orchestra. And just as the tuba should not drown out the flutes (since that ruins the overall effect), an overload of a single mineral doesn't play well within the body. The "too loud" mineral will compete with others for absorption, crowding them out and resulting in deficiencies of other vital substances. Too much calcium, for example, can result in a magnesium deficiency. And too much copper can crowd out zinc. That's why it's important to balance your dosages. If you "overdose" on one mineral, you're probably headed for a deficiency in another.

Having warned you, I can now tell you that taking mineral supplements may be tremendously beneficial to you, the PMS sufferer. Magnesium, in particular, is often low in those who suffer from PMS, and just eating magnesium-rich foods and taking a magnesium supplement may help turn the tide on estrogen dominance, water retention, menstrual migraines, and sugar cravings. But to avoid overloading on one mineral or another, buy a multimineral (or multivitamin/mineral) that contains the kinds and amounts of minerals listed below.

CALCIUM

What it does in general: Calcium keeps bones and teeth strong and healthy, helps maintain proper blood pressure, and aids in muscle contraction, transmission of nerve signals, and various enzyme systems. It also helps prevent irregular heartbeat, muscle cramps, insomnia, depression, high blood pressure, osteoporosis, and cognitive impairment.

How it can ease PMS: Studies have shown that calcium supplements can help ease water retention, food cravings, mood swings, headaches, and pain in PMS sufferers. It can also quell anxiety, nervousness, and joint pain. In 1998, a research team out of St. Luke's Roosevelt Hospital in New York performed a study of 466 women with moderate-to-severe PMS symptoms, including pain, mood swings, food cravings, and water retention. The women were divided into two groups, with one receiving a daily 1,200 mg calcium supplement, the other a placebo. After three months, those who were taking the calcium supplement had 48 percent fewer overall symptoms of PMS, while those who got the placebo had only a 30 percent reduction in symptoms.

   Why? No one is quite sure why calcium can help relieve PMS. Undoubtedly, its anti-inflammatory effects and the role it plays in the production of serotonin are part of the equation. Some also theorize that when calcium levels in the body fall too low, hormones are released that fire up the symptoms of PMS.

Recommended Dosage for PMS: For the general population, it's typically recommended that calcium and magnesium be taken in a 2:1 ratio (for example, 1,200 mg calcium and 600 mg magnesium). But since magnesium deficiency is so widespread among PMS sufferers, many PMS experts recommend that the ratio be reversed: that is, twice as much magnesium as calcium. Since the jury is still out on this, you may find a 1:1 ratio the safest way to go—say 400 mg of each. The best kind of calcium supplement to take is calcium citrate because it's easily absorbed and doesn't appear to contribute to the development of kidney stones.

Food sources: Dairy products (use the nonfat kind), canned salmon or sardines (you'll need to eat the bones), oysters, calcium-fortified soy milk, calcium-fortified orange juice, spinach, collard greens, tofu, and almonds. Be aware, however, that the calcium found in vegetables is often poorly absorbed by the body, due to fiber and certain other substances contained in plants.

MAGNESIUM

What it does in general: Magnesium plays a vital role in many of the body's metabolic processes. It's needed to convert fat, carbohydrates, and protein into energy, and to regulate heartbeat, blood sugar, muscle contraction/relaxation, nerve impulses, and the electrical balance within the cells. Magnesium works in conjunction with calcium to perform many of these functions, so a deficiency in magnesium will affect calcium metabolism, as well.

How it can ease PMS: Magnesium helps the liver deactivate estrogen. It also helps reduce water retention, improve glucose tolerance, and ease menstrual migraines. A lack of magnesium can cause migraine headaches, mood swings, sugar cravings, cramps or muscle spasms, irregular heartbeat, weakened bones, osteoporosis, fluid retention, fatigue, and low energy.

Most women have low magnesium levels during the premenstrual phase, but those with PMS often have extra-low levels. A lack of sufficient magnesium can result from estrogen excess, stress, alcohol, pregnancy, heavy exercise, diarrhea, vomiting, diabetes, old age, and excessive calcium intake. Luckily, magnesium supplements seem to help. In one study, women with PMS who were given 360 mg of magnesium three times a day showed a significant decrease in symptoms after taking the mineral for just two months.

Another study showed a significant reduction in water retention in PMS sufferers who took 200 mg of magnesium oxide every day throughout two cycles.

Recommended Dosage for PMS: Only about 25 percent of Americans meet the RDA for magnesium, which is 350 mg. Many PMS experts recommend even larger doses—say, 400–800 mg. You may want to start at a lower dose, however, since too much magnesium can cause diarrhea. Begin by taking 200 mg, then increase to 400 mg after a few weeks if your body seems to tolerate it well. When you reach the 400 mg level, take the magnesium in divided doses (e.g., 200 mg in the morning and 200 mg in the evening). It's better absorbed and more easily tolerated that way. Then, if you wish, gradually increase your dose over a period of weeks to a maximum of 800 mg per day, reducing the dosage if diarrhea occurs. Taking magnesium in the form of *magnesium oxide* may help ease water retention, while *magnesium aspartate* may help reduce fatigue.

Food sources: Wheat bran, wheat germ, whole-wheat flour, nuts, beans, peas, dark-green leafy vegetables, dried apricots, fish, and tofu.

ZINC

What it does in general: Zinc is present in every cell of the body and is a vital part of more than two hundred enzymes. It's a component of many of the body's hormones, including insulin, the sex hormones, and thyroid hormones, and also plays an important part in immune function.

How it can ease PMS: Zinc deficiency, which can be brought about by estrogen excess, can cause increased production of the inflammation-producing prostaglandins. As a result, estrogen levels can be pushed even higher, suppressing the action of progesterone, and kicking off the production of cortisol. Taking in adequate amounts of zinc, then, can help restore balance to your hormones, support progesterone production, decrease excess estrogen, and aid in the production of the "good" kind of prostaglandins, which ease inflammation. Zinc also helps stimulate the immune system and control acne.

Recommended Dosage for PMS: 25–50 mg

Food sources: Oysters, seafood, liver, eggs, whole grains, dried beans, and peas.

BORON

What it does in general: Boron plays a major role in calcium and magnesium metabolism. It helps the body "hold on" to these minerals, rather than losing them through the urine. (Even if you get plenty of calcium in your diet, if you don't have enough boron, you may excrete enough calcium and/or magnesium to seriously weaken your bones.) Boron also helps increase mental alertness and enhance brain function. Typically, this mineral is used to prevent or treat osteoporosis and/or arthritis.

How it can ease PMS: Because it reduces the excretion of calcium and magnesium (two minerals that are vital for preventing and controlling PMS), boron may help ease migraine headaches, mood swings, water retention, sugar cravings, and other effects of calcium and/or magnesium deficiency.

Recommended Dosage for PMS: 3–9 mg

Food sources: Fruits and vegetables, particularly apples, peaches, pears, grapes, legumes, almonds, and peanuts.

IODINE

What it does in general: Iodine is necessary for good thyroid function and regulation of metabolism. It has an antibiotic effect, guards against toxicity from radiation, and is needed for wound healing and maintenance of skin, hair, and nails. It also boosts immune function and prevents the buildup of mucus.

How it can ease PMS: An iodine deficiency can result in menstrual difficulties and PMS. That's because *thyroxine*, the thyroid hormone that regulates the metabolic rate, helps control estrogen levels. If you don't get enough iodine, your thyroid gland can't produce enough thyroxine, and that means that your estrogen levels can start to build up.

Recommended Dosage for PMS: The RDA for iodine is 150 mcg. The most obvious source of iodine is iodized salt, but since you're trying to avoid added salt, look to kelp, seaweed, or other food sources of iodine, instead.

An easy way of ensuring that you're getting enough iodine is by taking 1,000–1,500 mg of kelp in supplement form. You can also take six to eight iodine drops mixed into a glass of water, but check with your doctor first and get your thyroid levels checked. If you're in the normal range, it's probably best to take a multimineral that contains the RDA of 150 mcg although some people have enjoyed good results at 250 mcg. Ask your doctor.

Food sources: Iodized salt, seafood, kelp, saltwater fish, seaweed, sesame seeds, asparagus, garlic, soybeans, turnip greens, and Swiss chard.

CHROMIUM

What it does in general: Chromium is an important element in the control of blood glucose levels, working with insulin to help get glucose, the body's fuel, into the cells. Unfortunately, just about everybody is deficient in this mineral and, to make matters worse, chromium levels decrease with age. This may explain why we've seen such a rise in obesity and Type II diabetes in recent years, as we eat more and more, but feel less and less satisfied. Decreasing chromium levels may also play a part in the development of heart disease. Chromium supplements are typically used to treat hypo-glycemia, diabetes, high cholesterol, weight problems, elevated triglycerides, and acne.

How it can ease PMS: If you've got trouble with low blood sugar—sugar cravings or other food cravings, irritability, fatigue, increased appetite, etc.—you probably need to get more chromium in your diet. Chromium may help prevent both the skyrocketing of blood sugar and its evil twin, hypoglycemia.

Recommended Dosage for PMS: 200–400 mcg of chromium pico-linate, the most absorbable form of chromium.

Food sources: The best food sources of chromium are liver and other organ meats, brewer's yeast, nuts, and whole grains. It's difficult to get enough from diet alone, so you'll probably need to take a supplement.

PUTTING IT ALL TOGETHER

I recommend the following minerals to help combat PMS:

Boron	3–9 mg
Calcium	400 mg
Chromium	200–400 mcg
Iodine	250 mcg
Magnesium	400 mg
Zinc	25–50 mg

You'll probably be able to get most of these (plus all of the vitamins listed in the previous chapter) in a good multi-vitamin/multi-mineral supplement. You may need to take a few additional supplements to meet the above recommendations, but try to keep it as simple as possible. (Besides being complicated, it gets expensive!) The simpler your supplement regimen and the fewer pills you have to take, the more likely you'll be to stick with it.

11

Get Up and Exercise!

You already know (I'm sure!) that exercise is an absolute *must* for any-one who wants to build and maintain good health. That's because regular exercise strengthens your heart and lungs, improves your cir-culation, lowers your blood pressure, and decreases your levels of cir-culating blood fats, a major contributor to heart disease. Exercise also builds your muscles, increases your stamina, and improves your bal-ance—which enhances your overall physical abilities and makes it less likely that you'll become injured. As if that weren't enough, it also revs up your immune system, improves your looks, and gives your sex drive a boost.

WHAT EXERCISE CAN DO FOR PMS

But did you know that exercise also helps prevent or relieve PMS? It does. Studies have shown that athletes, dancers, and other women who are in good physical condition have fewer and milder symptoms of PMS. Regular exercise is particularly helpful in relieving symptoms related to depression and tension, such as mood swings, fatigue, irri-tability, and cramps. For maximum benefits, experts recommend at least twenty minutes of exercise (preferably aerobic) every day, particularly during the premenstrual phase. That's because exercise can help:

- **Reduce water retention**—Exercise gets bodily fluids moving, thus reducing congestion in the female organs and easing abdominal bloating. Excess water is "sweated out," relieving water retention and swelling.
- **Oxygenate the body**—Many women tend to hunch their shoulders, collapsing the chest and "doubling up" in response to pain. They also take shallow breaths, which means that less oxygen is delivered to the tissues and toxic substances start to build up. But exercise encourages deep breathing, which improves circulation and brings plenty of oxygen to the tissues. At the same time, exercise improves the posture and strengthens the muscles and connective tissues, taking excess pressure off organs and joints and relieving pain.
- **Relieve muscle tension**—Exercise is one of the world's best antidotes to stress-induced tension and tightness in the muscles. If you're feeling all "knotted up" after a hard day's work, a good workout may be one of the best stress-relieving techniques in the world. Besides loosening up the muscles and reducing tension, exercise helps burn off stress hormones and lowers pain levels.
- **Increase the feeling of well-being**—Your body produces extra endorphins, the "feel good" hormones, in response to exercise, which help improve your mood, relieve depression, block pain, and increase your sense of well-being.
- **Reduce mental and emotional stress levels**—Exercise releases mental tension, while also easing anxiety, nervousness, hostility, and irritability.
- **Improve the quality of sleep**—On the days that you work out, you'll probably find that you fall asleep more easily and sleep more deeply.
- **Increase your overall energy level**—In general, you'll find that you have more energy once you've been exercising regularly. This is probably due to a combination of factors: less overall muscle tension

dragging you down, increased endorphin levels, muscles that work more efficiently, decreased levels of stress hormones, better quality sleep, etc.

BUT TAKE IT EASY . . . ESPECIALLY AT FIRST

With all of these potential benefits, running the gamut from mood stabilization to increased relaxation to improved energy, you'd be crazy not to include exercise in your arsenal of weapons against PMS. But before you throw on your running shoes and go for a ten-mile jog, be sure to see your physician to make sure your body can handle it. Then, instead of plunging into exercise whole hog, begin slowly with mild exercise, especially if you haven't done anything in a long time. Walk instead of run, swim at an easy pace instead of a frantic one, and cycle on flat ground instead of heading for the hills. Then, once you've built some strength and stamina, go ahead and increase both the length and intensity of your workout—but, again, gradually.

THE ELEMENTS OF A GOOD EXERCISE PLAN

You can exercise in a million different ways: walking, running, dancing, practicing karate, joining an aerobics class, doing tai chi, wrestling, or even flinging yourself around the uneven parallel bars. But exercise is most effective when it's part of a plan, and any good exercise plan includes five basic elements:

Warm-Up

You should always spend at least ten minutes at the beginning of your workout session doing mild warm-up exercises to get your circulation going and to raise the temperature in your muscles. Jumping jacks, slow jogging, brisk walking, jumping rope, or doing light calisthenics will get your body in the right mode for movement and help prevent injuries.

Cardiovascular Endurance Exercises

You probably know this form of exercise as "aerobics," but you don't have to join a class in order to do cardiovascular endurance exercises. Anything that speeds up your heart rate and makes you breathe more deeply and rapidly will qualify, including fast-paced walking, jogging, running, cycling, and continuous dancing. These are great for strengthening your heart, increasing the capacity of your lungs, and burning up excess fat. This form of exercise is particularly important for PMS control, since it stimulates sweating, relieves muscle tension, burns up stress hormones, and stimulates endorphin release.

Strengthening Exercises

Strengthening exercises help your muscles increase the force they can exert (strength) and the amount of time that they can exert that force (endurance). They help build and tone not only your muscles, but also your bones, tendons, and ligaments. An important element in strengthening exercises is the principle of resistance. Your muscles must work against something that either pushes or pulls against them, whether in the form of weights, gravity, water, or another part of your own body. Weight lifting, swimming, leg lifts, push-ups, and isometric exercises (i.e. placing your palms together and pushing) are all examples of strengthening exercises.

Stretching

These exercises will increase your ability to bend, twist, and reach, thereby improving your overall flexibility. Stretching makes your muscles more elastic and increases the range of motion of your joints, making your muscles, tendons, ligaments, and joints more resistant to injury. Stretching is also a great way to relieve stress, ease muscle pain, and increase relaxation, all of which are beneficial in the war against PMS. Stretching should always be done slowly and carefully to avoid injuring the muscles and the connective tissue. When you assume a stretching position, stretch as far as you can comfortably, then hold it there for thirty to forty-five seconds. Do *not* bounce (pull and release within the stretch). Toward the end of the time frame, try to stretch just a little farther, hold for a few seconds, then slowly release. There are few things as relaxing as a good stretching session. But be careful. Take the time to learn the correct ways to stretch from a trained professional, for if you stretch incorrectly, you can end up doing more harm than good.

Cool-Down

This is quite a bit like the warm-up session (you can do the very same exercises, if you wish), but the goal is just the opposite. Instead of revving up the body, you now want to decelerate. Gradually slow your pace and let your body know that it's time to go back down to its normal cruising speed. Don't exercise at full tilt and then stop suddenly. Think of yourself as a racehorse. You need to be walked around the track a few times before you go back to grazing in the field.

PUTTING THE ELEMENTS TOGETHER

To construct your own individualized fitness plan, apply these principles, no matter what kind of exercise you like to do:

- Warm up for at least ten minutes at the beginning of your session. Ideally, you won't move on to the rest of your exercise program until you've broken a sweat. Do not do stretches as a warm-up. They don't increase your heart rate, and your muscles can be injured when they're stretched cold.

- For maximum benefit, cardiovascular-endurance exercises should be done for twenty to thirty consecutive minutes, three times a week. You may want to start with ten-minute sessions, or even five-minute sessions, if you find that longer exercise periods are too exhausting. Then gradually increase the length of your cardiovascular workouts over time. A good goal would be a five-minute increase every week or two until you reach twenty to thirty minutes per session.
- Strengthening exercises should be done on the days you don't do cardio exercises (for example, strengthening on Monday, Wednesday, Friday; cardio on Tuesday, Thursday, Saturday). Start with ten- to fifteen-minute sessions and gradually build up to twenty to thirty minutes. Always work carefully and add resistance gradually so you don't strain or injure yourself. You may need to be supervised by a professional trainer, at least in the beginning.
- Stretching exercises should become part of your daily routine, performed ideally for about ten to twenty minutes. Do some overall stretches and then zero in on a different area of your body each day (i.e., shoulder stretches today, hip stretches tomorrow). Stretch only after you're thoroughly warmed up. The best time to stretch is at the end of your cardio or strengthening workout.
- Don't forget to cool down! Take five to ten minutes to bring your body back down to its usual speed by walking slowly, stretching, and doing some deep breathing.

What's the best exercise in the world for relieving the symptoms of PMS? Why, the kind you'll actually do on a regular basis, of course! Walking briskly around the park every day is better than doing a two-hour workout at the gym once a week. Find some form of movement that you really enjoy, then do it—regularly!

12

Natural Progesterone

Many women have achieved excellent relief from PMS symptoms through the use of natural progesterone, which has become one of today's fastest-rising "stars" in the treatment of menstrual problems. Since too much estrogen (the nemesis of progesterone) and too little progesterone appear to be the cause of PMS in as many as 75 percent of its victims, giving supplementary progesterone to these women certainly seems to make sense. The hormone can ease a multitude of PMS symptoms including:

- mood swings
- irritability
- depression
- anxiety
- breast tenderness
- water retention
- weight gain
- sluggish thyroid
- insomnia

But even though it seems to be the "latest thing," progesterone therapy is not a new idea. Way back in the 1940s a British gynecologist named Katherina Dalton began experimenting with high-dose progesterone suppositories as a treatment for PMS (a syndrome that she herself first defined). Since that time, with dosages adjusted and methods refined, progesterone has proved to be an effective treatment not only for PMS, but also for menopausal symptoms, fibrocystic breast disease, endometriosis, menstrual migraines, and ovarian cysts, among other conditions.

In the early days of progesterone therapy, the hormone was either given by injection or in suppository form, but today it's also available as a cream, in capsule or sublingual (under the tongue) form, as a liquid, or as a vaginal or rectal suppository. Typically, progesterone replacement is administered during the phase when the body would normally produce the hormone on its own: beginning, say, any time from Day Ten to Day Fifteen and ending about Day Twenty-Eight (or the last day before menstruation). No progesterone is taken during the first two weeks of the cycle when the body normally produces very little of the hormone (from the first day of menstruation to Day Fourteen, the day that ovulation typically occurs). By applying progesterone in this on-and-off pattern, you can mimic the body's normal cycle of progesterone production—which is important, especially when you're trying to balance your hormone levels.

NATURAL VERSUS SYNTHETIC

There's plenty of confusion about the difference between natural progesterone and synthetic progesterone. One friend of mine insisted that progesterone in any form other than the topical cream (i.e., pills, capsules, suppositories, etc.) had to be synthetic because it was obviously manufactured in the laboratory. But the terms "natural" and "synthetic" refer to the chemical structure of the progesterone, not the fact that it's in pill or cream form. Natural progesterone, no matter which way it's presented, has the exact same chemical "shape" as the progesterone in your body. If your own progesterone were in the shape of a key, for example, natural progesterone would be an exact copy of that key.

Synthetic progesterone, on the other hand, would be a slightly different key. It's not found in your body or anywhere else in nature—it can only be manufactured in a lab. Both the natural and the synthetic keys will fit into the progesterone receptor sites on your cells and turn the lock. Both, then, will be allowed entry into the cell, and both will exert certain hormonal effects. For example, both natural and synthetic progesterone will oppose estrogen, helping to keep estrogen dominance in check. Both will also protect against cancer of the lining of the uterus and aid in the formation of new bone. But since the synthetic version is not an exact copy of natural progesterone, it can't provide all of the benefits of natural progesterone. For example, natural progesterone will aid in thyroid function, protect against breast cancer, help normalize the fatty-acid profile, assist in restoration of normal sex drive, and help regulate sleep patterns.

Synthetic progesterone, in contrast, can provide none of these benefits and, instead, contributes some out-and-out detriments. To start with, it interferes with your body's production of its own natural progesterone and competes for receptor sites with the progesterone that you do manage to manufacture. Both of these actions effectively reduce your levels of this important hormone. To make matters worse, the use of synthetic progesterone can cause several unpleasant side effects including mood swings, tiredness, depression, abdominal bloating, breast tenderness, weight gain, muscle or joint pain, dry skin, dry eyes, acne, and anxiety. So taking synthetic progesterone to relieve PMS can be a lot like hitting yourself in the head to relieve a headache! Natural progesterone, on the other hand, functions just like real progesterone in your body, helping to smooth out mood swings, ease water retention and breast tenderness, stimulate a sluggish thyroid, and improve sleep.

Synthetic forms of progesterone (also known as progestins) are manufactured from either natural progesterone or testosterone.

They're typically found in birth control pills and various forms of hormone replacement therapy under generic names like hydroxy-progesterone, medroxyprogesterone, megestrol, norethindrone, and norgestrel. (Brand names include Provera, Depo-Provera, and Megace.) Natural progesterone comes from a substance found in wild yams or soybeans that's converted to progesterone that is identical to the progesterone produced in the body. (The generic name is simply "progesterone"; brand names include Prometrium, Pro-Gest, and Crinone.)

ORAL PROGESTERONE VERSUS THE CREAM

Natural progesterone comes in several forms, among them the capsule, topical cream (rubbed on the skin), vaginal suppository, and sublingual drops (placed under the tongue). Which is best? Many experts recommend the topical cream because it's easily absorbed, it's gradually released into the system in a way that mimics the ovaries' natural release of progesterone, and, perhaps most importantly, it doesn't produce anywhere near as many progesterone metabolites (breakdown products).

You see, when you take oral progesterone (pills), even though it's natural, about 90 percent of what you take ends up as breakdown products. That's because the progesterone must first pass through your intestines and into the liver, where the majority of it is "chewed up" and sent through the bloodstream on its way to being excreted. But all of this "junk" floating through your bloodstream has some undesirable effects. Some of it will take up residence in your progesterone receptor sites, crowding out the progesterone you really need. Because of this, you can wind up becoming less sensitive to progesterone and less able to receive its benefits. Over time, the buildup of these breakdown products puts a strain on your liver and can also cause changes in brain function, resulting in depression and memory problems.

Suppositories and sublingual drops don't result in an overload of breakdown products, but they tend to make progesterone levels rise very quickly, then recede. This causes a sort of hormonal roller-coaster effect that's unlike the body's natural, more gradual pattern of progesterone release.

The topical creams, however, don't have either of these problems. They don't go through the digestive system, so they aren't immediately broken down in the liver and excreted. Because of this, much smaller doses can be taken (15–30 mg as opposed to the oral dose of 100–400 mg). The level of breakdown products, then, is much lower and the metabolites are easily excreted, so there is no buildup effect. And the delivery system is much more natural. When the cream is applied to the skin, the progesterone first makes its way into the fat layer just underneath the skin where it is gradually released into the bloodstream in amounts that approximate the normal levels of progesterone in the body.

WHAT KIND OF CREAM AND HOW MUCH?

There are many brands of progesterone cream, some of which are available by prescription only and others that are available over the counter. Beware of the over-the-counter versions, though, since it may be hard to gauge just how much progesterone you're getting. And watch out for any that contain "wild yam extract," "diosgenin," or "Dioscorea," all of which are names for the substance that's extracted from wild yams and converted into natural progesterone. While this substance is identical to your natural progesterone *once it's been converted in a lab*, the plain, unconverted stuff is useless as a progesterone source. So make sure you're getting the real thing, not just the raw material.

It's safer to get your doctor to write you a prescription for a natural progesterone cream, one that can be made especially for you by a compounding pharmacy. John R. Lee, M.D., author of *What Your Doctor May Not Tell You About Premenopause* and an expert on the topic of natural progesterone, suggests that you use a 1.6 percent cream containing 450–500 mg of progesterone per ounce. The cream should not contain mineral oil, since that will block the skin's absorption of the progesterone. It should also be free of herbs, phytoestrogens, and synthetic progesterone.

Dr. Lee suggests that you use as much as two full ounces of this cream throughout a sixteen- to eighteen-day period, beginning on Day Ten or Twelve and ending on Day Twenty-Six or Thirty. Twice a day (morning and evening), rub ⅛–½ teaspoon on an area of your body where the skin is soft and hairless, like the insides of your upper arms, the neck, the chest area, the palms of the hands or the soles of the feet (unless calloused). Rotate your application areas—use a different area each time. Dr. Lee also suggests that you use a "crescendo pattern," beginning with smaller dabs (⅛ tsp.) on Days Ten to Twelve, then gradually increasing to larger doses (½ tsp.) on the days just before your period, when you'll use up the remainder of your two ounces. If your PMS symptoms seem to subside after trying this regimen for a few months, reduce the amount of progesterone cream you use to one ounce (one-half container), and see if you still get good results. Adjust, if necessary.

A BALANCING ACT

It's important to remember that everybody is different and every *body* is different. The tricky thing about female hormones is that they're in a constant state of flux, which makes them hard to measure. You can ask for a blood test, but that will only give you a "snapshot" of what your hormonal levels are at that particular moment. Things may have been different an hour before the test, just as they may be an hour later. Your best gauge of whether or not your hormones are in balance is how you feel. If you're anxious, nervous, irritable, blown up like a balloon from water retention, and feel like you could eat an entire one-pound box of chocolates all by yourself, you're probably suffering from estrogen dominance and could benefit from a little natural progesterone. But if you start taking progesterone and find yourself sleepy, lethargic, mildly depressed, and suffering from breast tenderness, you're probably taking too much and need to cut back a little. It's a delicate balancing act, and you'll need to pay strict attention to your body's signals in order to make it work.

13

Herbs

For thousands of years, herbs were our primary medicines. We used them for all kinds of "female problems," including the pain, bloating, and other symptoms of PMS. Herbs are still used for these reasons today, even though most modern physicians don't consider them to be viable treatments. But herbs *can* function as medicines, albeit gentle ones, unlike our formidable modern drugs. Instead of overpowering the symptoms, as drugs do, herbs offer the body the tools it needs to regain balance and heal itself. Numerous herbs can be used for PMS; some to alleviate pain, others to reduce bloating, still others to ease anxiety, and so on. I could write an entire book just on herbs for PMS. Unfortunately, we don't have enough space to include all of the information here, so I'll just mention ten of my favorites.

BLACK COHOSH (*Cimifuga racemosa*)

Black cohosh has a long history, dating back to Native Americans who used it as an aid for menstrual problems, labor, and childbirth. They named it *cohosh*, which means "rough," because its roots were rough.

European settlers soon adopted this herb, and it became a prime ingredient in their "Vegetable Compound," a popular tonic for women's problems in nineteenth-century America.

With the advent of modern pharmaceuticals in the twentieth century, black cohosh was relegated to the back of the medicine chest. But it became popular again in the latter part of the century, as we learned more about its properties.

Black cohosh has estrogen-like actions that appear to "re-balance" female hormones. Because it has the ability to occupy estrogen receptor sites, while exerting just a weak estrogenic action, it can actually lower high estrogen levels and reduce the effects of estrogen dominance. In women who are lacking in estrogen, black cohosh can supply a mild estrogenic boost. And because it slows the secretion of luteinizing hormone (LH), it's also helpful for reducing several of the symptoms of menopause. Black cohosh is used to relax the muscles and ease headaches, pain, and muscle spasms. It also has an anti-inflammatory effect, and it is helpful in relieving stress and nervous tension.

Black cohosh has not received any official recognition in the United States, but in Germany the scientific board responsible for evaluating herbal remedies has stated that it's a safe and effective approach to relieving the symptoms of PMS, other menstrual disorders, and the symptoms of menopause.

There is no set dosage of black cohosh; some experts recommend drinking ten to twenty-five drops of black cohosh extract mixed in liquid or taking up to 40 mg in capsule form per day. You'll also find the herb in various formulas, sometimes in combination with blue cohosh.

Black cohosh is nontoxic and generally considered to be safe. However, it should not be used during pregnancy, especially in the early stages, for it can stimulate the uterus and bring on premature contractions.

CHAMOMILE (*Matricaria chamomilla*)

Although chamomile tea is used primarily for its relaxing qualities, the herb exerts a number of other positive effects on the body, due to its natural anti-inflammatory, antibacterial, and antifungal ingredients.

Chamomile has been used for hundreds of years to treat insomnia, back pain, arthritis, and other ailments, including "female anxiety." Today, herbalists recommend it for soothing PMS symptoms triggered by tension or stress. It's also an antispasmodic (good for relieving cramps and other gynecologic complaints) and helps support the action of both the liver and the digestive system.

Although there is no set dosage for chamomile, many experts suggest drinking a cup of chamomile tea (made from one tablespoon of chamomile flowers steeped in a cup of boiling water) three times daily, or drinking ten to twenty drops of extract mixed with water two to three times a day.

WARNING: Those who are allergic to ragweed, chrysanthemums, or other members of the aster or daisy families may have a reaction to chamomile. If you want to try this herb, start with the smallest possible dose and watch for adverse effects.

CHASTE TREE BERRY (*Vitex agnus-castus*)

During the Middle Ages, monks used the dried, ripened berry of the chaste tree (sometimes referred to as *monk's berry*) to quell their sexual desire—thus the reference to chastity.

Today we know that chaste tree berry extract (also known as Vitex or VACE) helps to balance your hormones by binding to dopamine receptors in the pituitary gland. This, in turn, reduces your production of prolactin. Because prolactin and progesterone tend to counterbalance each other, reducing prolactin boosts your progesterone

levels. And as progesterone levels rise, the symptoms of PMS generally decrease, especially in women with estrogen dominance. (Sure
enough, researchers have found that those with PMS tend to have
higher-than-normal prolactin levels throughout their cycles, particularly in the second and third weeks.)

The combined results of three large studies (a total of 4,500
women) on the effect of chaste tree berry extract on PMS are excit-
ing. At a daily dosage of forty to forty-two drops of liquid extract
(equivalent to 30–40 mg of crude plant extract), nearly one-third of
the women reported complete relief from PMS symptoms, while more
than half reported marked improvement.

The average dose of chaste tree berry contains the equivalent of
20–40 mg of the crude plant extract (a maximum of forty-two drops
of liquid extract). Or, if you want to take the tincture (a concoction
in which the herb has been steeped in alcohol), try ½ teaspoon before
breakfast over a period of several months. But don't take chaste tree
berry in conjunction with birth control pills, since its antagonistic
effects on prolactin can end up decreasing the pill's contraceptive
action. Also, avoid this herb if you're pregnant.

WARNING: Chaste tree berry extract has been known to cause ovarian hyperstimulation syndrome, so consult your doctor before taking it.

DANDELION (*Taraxacum officinale*)

Yes, the same annoying weed that pops up constantly amid the grass
in your lawn is actually a highly nutritious herb that can help you fight
certain symptoms of PMS! Loaded with beta-carotene, vitamin C,
iron, calcium, potassium, and other minerals, the dandelion is an
excellent diuretic that helps the body shed the excess water responsible for both menstrual bloating and breast tenderness.

Dandelion also contains two starch-like substances called levulin and inulin that help stabilize blood glucose levels. And the herb is known for stimulating and supporting liver function, which is vital in the breakdown and elimination of old estrogen. Constipation, headaches, and acne may also be eased through the use of this herb.

Virtually the entire dandelion plant—flowers, leaves, and roots—can be used for herbal treatment. Tea can be made from the roots or leaves, juice can be extracted from the plant, and the leaves can be eaten either raw or cooked. Tinctures and extracts are also available at health-food stores.

There is no set dosage for dandelion; some experts suggest taking ten to thirty drops of dandelion extract mixed with liquid every day. However if you eat fresh dandelion greens instead, you'll also be getting vitamins, minerals, levulin, inulin, fiber, and all of the other helpful substances that are in this herb, not just those that have been extracted.

DONG QUAI (*Angelica sinensis*)

Sometimes called "the female ginseng," dong quai has long been used to relieve a variety of female ailments, including menstrual cramps, irregular menstrual cycles, PMS, and the symptoms of menopause. An enormously popular herb, dong quai may help regulate and normalize the production and use of female hormones. Like black cohosh, it contains compounds that exert a mild estrogenic effect and compete with the body's estrogen for receptor sites. As a result, it can increase low levels of estrogen or decrease high levels. Dong quai also helps strengthen the actions of the liver and endocrine systems and exerts a calming, relaxing effect on the nervous system.

There are no set dosages for this herb, so you'll have to experiment and see what works best for you. You should not take this herb during menstruation or while pregnant. Take a small dosage (say, one capsule three times a day) beginning one week before your period is due, then continue to take it until menses begin. Repeat one week before your next cycle. The active ingredients in dong quai are found in the root, which can be chopped, sliced, or grated, and made into tea. It is also available as a tincture, extract, or powder.

FALSE UNICORN ROOT (*Chamaelirium luteum*)

This herb, a favorite of Native Americans, is known as an excellent tonic for the reproductive system, one that can normalize hormonal function and restore balance. That's because it contains hormone-like substances called *saponins* that exert a mild estrogenic effect. Thus, if you're low in estrogen, they'll boost your levels. And if you've got too much estrogen, they'll lower your levels of this hormone by blocking some of the estrogen receptor sites on the cell membranes. False unicorn root is believed to be an antidote to all uterine problems, including delayed menstrual periods, and may also ease migraine headaches.

Some experts recommend that one to two teaspoons of the grated root be simmered in one cup of water for ten to fifteen minutes, then sipped three times a day. Or, 2–4 ml of the tincture may be taken mixed in a glass of water three times a day.

MILK THISTLE (*Silybum marianum*)

Support for the liver is very important in the control of PMS, since this detoxifying organ plays a major role in the breakdown and excretion of old, used estrogen. The liver also detoxifies harmful substances such as alcohol, pollutants, and nicotine, transforming them into more benign substances that can pass through the body without wreaking total havoc. Milk thistle helps enhance liver function and produce new liver cells, owing to the action of *silymarin*, a flavonoid that strengthens the liver at the cellular level. Not only does milk thistle support general liver function, it also increases the level of *glutathione*, a powerful antioxidant, and aids in the breakdown of fats.

Milk thistle is available in capsule form (make sure it contains at least 70 percent silymarin). It's recommended that one 140 mg capsule of milk thistle be taken as often as three times a day to support the liver and aid in the detoxification process.

MOTHERWORT (*Leonurus cardiaca*)

This herb's two names give clues as to its uses. Its common name, *motherwort*, indicates that it's an herb (wort) useful to mothers and other women. And its scientific name, *Leonurus cardiaca*, tells you that it can also be used for certain heart (cardiac) ailments.

Way back in the seventeenth century, motherwort was highly regarded as a tonic for difficult menstruation and labor. Nicholas Culpepper, a seventeenth-century herbalist, wrote that motherwort " . . . settles mothers' wombs and is a wonderful help to women in their sore travail [childbirth] . . . it also provoketh women's courses [the menstrual period]." Today, motherwort is used to bring on delayed menstruation, ease menstrual cramps, lessen water retention, soothe nervous tension, and generally ease the symptoms of PMS.

There is no set dosage of motherwort. Some experts recommend drinking ten to fifteen drops of motherwort extract mixed in liquid, three times a day. You can also use dried motherwort to make tea, taking one cup every day.

WARNING: Motherwort can cause the uterus to contract and is sometimes used to encourage labor, so it should not be used during pregnancy.

NETTLE (*Urtica dioica*)

Although you may shrink at the idea of having anything to do with the nettle, a plant that stings like crazy and causes painful red welts, this versatile herb has been used for centuries as an effective medicinal remedy. The ancient Greeks and Romans used the nettle to ease gout, rheumatism, and the bites of poisonous snakes and insects. They even used the fibers found in the nettle stalk as a basis for fabric. Nettles are also a nutritious and delicious food, as well as an excellent source of vitamins A, C, D, and K, calcium, iron, and chlorophyll.

For centuries, the nettle has been considered an excellent all-around tonic for women, used to help counteract PMS, excessive menstruation, hemorrhaging during childbirth, lack of milk production, and symptoms of menopause. Its use as an antidote to PMS is primarily due to its diuretic properties (easing water retention, bloating, and weight gain) and its high nutrient content, which can help counteract nutritional deficiencies. The symptoms of allergies, which are sometimes aggravated during the premenstrual phase, may also be reduced by taking either fresh or dried nettles.

You can take nettles as a tincture, as juice or tea, or in capsule form. You can also eat their freshly cooked greens. (Nettles are available at some health-food stores and gourmet markets). One to two teaspoons of the tincture, one or two ounces of the juice, two to three capsules, or a couple of cups of tea daily may be enough to achieve the desired results.

PENNYROYAL (*Hedeoma pulegioides*)

We don't know as much as we'd like to about this herb, which is sometimes called lung mint. It was used by the ancients as an insect repellant and for colds and flus, and was included in the *U.S. Pharmacopoeia* from the early nineteenth through the early twentieth centuries as a treatment for "women's problems" such as delayed menstruation. Native Americans used pennyroyal to ease menstrual cramps, and it's still used for that purpose today, as well as for relieving the bloating, breast tenderness, and tension that occur with PMS.

There is no set dosage of pennyroyal. Some authorities suggest drinking twenty to forty drops of extract mixed in liquid every day, or taking one tablespoon of dried pennyroyal herb mixed with water.

WARNING: Be careful with pennyroyal oil, as it's extremely toxic and doses as small as two teaspoons may cause convulsions or even death. Because it stimulates uterine contractions, pennyroyal oil can also trigger labor and should only be used under the supervision of a physician skilled in the use of herbs (and then only in limited amounts and for brief periods). The pennyroyal herb itself is considered much safer than its essential oil.

VALERIAN (*Valeriana officinalis*)

Noted for its calming effects on the body, valerian is often recommended to alleviate nervous tension, anxiety, and the effects of stress. An antispasmodic, valerian is used to ease cramps, muscle tension, and muscle pain, and is helpful as an antidote to high blood pressure and tension headaches. It may also aid in fighting depression, especially if it's caused by stress or nervous tension. Valerian is well known as a sleep aid; studies show that it can shorten the amount of time it takes to fall asleep, as well as increase sleep quality.

It's the root of the valerian plant that contains the active ingredients, and it can be taken in the form of extract, capsules, tinctures, or tea. To alleviate anxiety, some experts recommend a daily dose of ten drops of valerian extract mixed with water *or* taking one to two capsules two to three times a day *or* taking ½ teaspoon of tincture three times a day *or* drinking two to three cups of tea. For insomnia, take one of the following an hour before bedtime: fifteen drops of valerian extract mixed with water *or* two or three capsules *or* ¾ to 1 teaspoon of tincture *or* a couple of cups of tea.

IF YOU WANT TO TAKE HERBS . . .

Herbs should be taken with caution since they produce various effects on the body. Too much of any one herb, the wrong mixture of herbs, or the mixing of herbs and certain medications can be dangerous to your health. If you think you'd like to try herbal preparations to ease your PMS symptoms, visit a qualified herbalist and follow instructions. You should also consult with a medical doctor, especially if you have any medical conditions, are taking any medications that might be adversely affected by herbs, are pregnant or nursing, or intend to become pregnant soon.

14

Avoid Xenoestrogens

What do nail-polish remover, car exhaust, rubber cement, and feed-lot cattle have in common? They all contain substances called xeno-estrogens, chemicals that act like estrogen in your body and can worsen your PMS symptoms. Xenoestrogens (xeno is pronounced zee-no) are man-made substances that are structurally similar to estrogen, which gives them the ability to function like hormones within your body. You can think of the xenoestrogens as a stranger who somehow has gotten hold of a copy of your ATM card and your PIN number, and now has the ability to withdraw, deposit, or transfer your money as he sees fit. Even though he's not *you*, he can make certain things happen just as surely as you can.

XENOESTROGENS BRING ON ESTROGEN EXCESS

Known to disrupt hormone balance in both humans and animals, most xenoestrogens exert a feminizing effect on both male and female bodies, and experts say that these substances are at least partly responsible for our current epidemic of estrogen excess. Xenoestrogens help drive up estrogen levels by:

- Attaching to estrogen receptor sites and "acting" like estrogen.
- Encouraging the creation of brand-new estrogen receptor sites.
- Hampering the liver's ability to dismantle and excrete estrogen, increasing the estrogen "buildup" effect.

Just how these "fake" hormones can affect the body becomes apparent when you take a look at wildlife exposed to xenoestrogens. Male birds become sterile and their reproductive tracts start to resemble those of females, with ovarian tissue appearing in the testes. Turtles, mollusks, and fish actually switch from one gender to the next. Male alligators exposed to xenoestrogens develop abnormally small sex organs and extremely low testosterone levels; many become sterile. And a good percentage of the alligator eggs that are laid somehow never get around to hatching.

XENOESTROGENS AND THE OVARIES

Even more important may be the effects of xenoestrogens on the ovaries. When female animals are exposed to xenoestrogens while still in the womb, some of their follicles actually "burn out." As you may remember, it's the follicle that's responsible for making and housing the egg. Then, once the egg has popped out of the follicle and begun its journey through the fallopian tube, it's the discarded follicle that begins to produce progesterone. No follicle means no egg—and no progesterone. Many experts believe that our increasing incidences of progesterone deficiency and infertility could be the by-products of our exposure to xenoestrogens. The resulting hormonal imbalance may be responsible not only for our good friend PMS, but also for such wide-ranging effects as miscarriage, low sex drive, insomnia, fibrocystic breasts, water retention, mood disturbances, and an increased risk of breast, ovarian, or uterine cancers.

THE WORST OFFENDERS AND HOW TO AVOID THEM

If your PMS is due to estrogen excess, the last thing you need is to get another dose of estrogen from the environment. But even if you're estrogen deficient, you don't want *this* kind of estrogen clogging up your receptor sites, exerting a super-potent hormonal effect, and getting in the way of the good, natural estrogen that your body produces. So, do what you can to cut back or eliminate your exposure to the following:

• **Animal fats**—The fat that you get from meats, poultry, eggs, and dairy products most likely contains a high amount of xenoestrogens owing to the hormones, antibiotics, and pesticide-sprayed grains that domestic animals are routinely given to make them big, fat, and "healthy." Fish living in contaminated waters also contain xenoestrogens. Your best bet is to cut back or eliminate your intake of red meat, while eating limited amounts of nonfat dairy products and hormone-free poultry. Fish that come from fish farms are the safest, but they must have been fed plankton in order to be good sources of omega-3 fatty acids.

• **Petroleum products**—Unfortunately, you can't completely avoid exposure to these chemicals. Our world runs on gasoline, oil, diesel fuel, and other petroleum products, and they permeate our air, water, and soil. But you can achieve a certain amount of damage control. Stay inside on days when pollution is high, close the windows in your home, and use your air conditioner as a filter. While driving, roll up your car windows and use the car's air conditioner as a filter. Find a home that's as far away from traffic, factories, or other major sources of pollution as possible and don't inhale gasoline fumes when refilling your car. Also, minimize your exposure to solvents, glues, adhesives, or soaps made with petrochemical-based emulsifiers, as well as air fresheners, fabric softeners, and perfumed laundry soaps.

• **Plastics**—A major petrochemical by-product, plastics literally surround us as a major part of our furniture, packaging for our food and water, cooking and eating utensils, clothing, cars, appliances, electronics, etc. In general, the less exposure to plastics, the better, although you won't be able to replace everything with more natural products like wood or pottery. Try to avoid drinking water from plastic bottles and be particularly vigilant about not drinking hot beverages from plastic cups or microwaving foods in plastic containers, since some kinds of plastic will release xenoestrogens into the food or beverage when heated. (Use ceramic dishes or cups, instead.) Also, wear natural fibers instead of the plastic-based polyester or vinyl.

• **Aldehydes, alcohols**—Potent sources of xenoestrogens, the most likely culprits include nail polish and nail-polish remover. (Check out the list of chemicals on the package labels of these products!) If you can, stay away from aldehydes and alcohols, which are absorbed directly through the skin or nails into the fatty tissue below. (Try buffing your nails instead, for a nice, natural glow.)

• **Chlorine, chlorinated compounds**—Not only is chlorine a potent xenoestrogen, it also becomes carcinogenic at certain levels. Bleach, cleansers, and certain detergents are the main sources of chlorine in our environment. But you can easily avoid using them by making a paste of baking soda to use as a household scrub or filling a spray bottle with water plus a little white vinegar to clean windows, mirrors, and tile surfaces.

• **Nonylphenols**—These are by-products of the surfactants found in detergents (both laundry and dishwashing), cosmetics, pesticides, and herbicides that eventually wind up in our waterways in huge quantities. You may be familiar with nonoxynol-9, a common spermicide found in diaphragm jellies and condoms. (I bet you didn't realize you were applying a xenoestrogen directly to the sensitive walls of the vagina, where it is allowed to sit for anywhere from six to twenty-four hours!) To avoid nonylphenols, get rid of lawn sprays, bug sprays, flea removal products (collars, sprays, shampoos), and all other pesticides and herbicides. Buy only organically-grown, pesticide-free produce, use environmentally safe detergents, and stay away from spermicides. You'll be healthier and so will your environment.

- **Synthetic estrogens**—I suppose it goes without saying, but if you're trying to avoid xenoestrogens, don't turn around and take one of the biggest offenders of all—synthetic estrogen (i.e., man-made estrogen replacement and/or the birth control pill). Man-made estrogen is not only more potent than the kind your body makes, it functions differently within your body and can exert some serious potential side effects. If you and your doctor decide that you're estrogen deficient, opt for a form of natural estrogen replacement. As for birth control, find a non-chemical method.

15

Reduce Stress

Have you ever noticed that when you're really stressed, your PMS symptoms get even worse? Part of the reason is because stress actually eats up your progesterone and helps throw you into estrogen dominance! It works like this: when you're under stress, your body reacts the same way it would if you were suddenly confronted by a grizzly bear. Your heart starts to beat faster, your rate of breathing speeds up, your blood pressure increases, sugar is released into your bloodstream for quick energy and your muscles tense up. In short, your body prepares itself to do one of two things: either go into hand-to-hand combat with the bear (hand to paw?) or run like crazy! This state of mind (and of body) is known as the *stress response*. But several heavy-duty stress hormones have to be manufactured in order to get this response into gear. And they're manufactured at the expense of your progesterone supply.

STRESS AND PMS

The adrenal glands, two little hormone factories that sit atop the kidneys, play a big part in the stress response. When you're stressed, these glands release special stress hormones that send your body into overdrive. In order to speed up your body's ability to burn fuel and release amino acids to repair tissue damage, your body will start to pump out cortisol at about *twenty times* its normal rate! And guess what cortisol is made from? That's right, your very own progesterone. So your progesterone levels can take a nosedive when you're stressed, and if you're chronically stressed, you can find yourself in a permanent state of estrogen dominance. Cortisol also slows down your thyroid, which can bring on weight gain, fatigue, low sex drive, headaches, and certain other symptoms seen in PMS.

THE GOOD, THE BAD, AND THE UGLY

The body's ability to flood itself with stress hormones during emergencies is basic to survival. If you're in physical danger, you'll need to have the energy and the power to get yourself out of there! That's the good part about stress hormones.

Unfortunately, modern life stresses you in lots of ways that really *don't* require a physical response. In fact, a shower of stress hormones is probably the last thing you need when your boss starts yelling at you or somebody cuts you off in traffic, because you don't have a physical outlet for the big burst of energy that follows. Instead, you just have to sit there feeling your face get hot, your heart start to pound, and your hands start to shake from the rush of adrenaline. You certainly can't fight or flee, although your body is more than ready for either. There's nothing to do but sit there and stew in your own juices. That's the bad part about stress hormones.

And the ugly part is that chronic exposure to high levels of stress hormones is bad news for your body—bad for your heart, bad for your stomach, bad for your psychological health, and certainly bad for your hormonal balance. And yet you *need* those hormones, although you could probably live without them for a short time if you weren't stressed at all. Rats who have had their stress-hormone-producing adrenal glands removed can live perfectly healthy lives as long as they're fed nutritious foods and not subjected to stress. But once they become stressed, they die.

Does it seem like a case of can't live with 'em, can't live without 'em? It's not. You need to be able to produce stress hormones at times. But if your body is pumping them out at high levels all the time, your poor adrenal glands will eventually become exhausted and simply give out. And then you can find yourself suffering from debilitating fatigue, aches and pains, sugar cravings, allergies, and a weakened immune system. You can suffer the same fate if you're progesterone-deficient, since progesterone is the stuff from which the stress hormones are made. That's because too little progesterone results in a poor supply of stress hormones, making you weak, tired, and susceptible to disease.

USE YOUR STRESS HORMONES SPARINGLY

In short, you don't want to overspend your stress hormones. In order to save these precious hormones for real emergencies and to keep your adrenals from burning out, you need to distinguish between what's really an emergency and what isn't. Do you *really* need to prepare for war when someone cuts in front of you in line? Is it truly a *catastrophe* when your child brings home a B instead of an A on her report card? Do you *always* have to have the last word? In other words, rethink some of the things that get you going and try to put them in perspective. As they say, don't sweat the small stuff—and it's almost all small stuff.

DECOMPRESSING

Just changing your attitude can reduce some of the stress in your life, but you'll probably still have plenty left over. That's why it's important to find an "escape valve" for stress and tension, so it doesn't accumulate and make your PMS worse. One of the best all-around stress relievers is exercise, especially aerobic exercise and stretching. Both are great for relieving muscle tension, increasing endorphin levels, and relaxing the body. Deep breathing, meditating, yoga, tai chi, and prayer are also excellent ways to calm your body and mind, center yourself, and shut out the world. Warm baths, massage, aromatherapy, a good belly laugh, and anything else that helps you slow down, relax, and escape from the pressures of our fast-paced world are also highly recommended. (See the chapters to follow for more information on some of these relaxation techniques.) One thing I can guarantee: if you reduce your stress levels, you'll reduce your PMS.

16

Yoga

Yoga, a mainstay of the Indian system of healing called Ayurveda, has been practiced for thousands of years as a physical and mental discipline aimed at joining the body, mind, emotions, and spirit in a harmonious union. The name "yoga" comes from the Sanskrit word *yug*, which means "yoke" or "union," and originally this combination of gentle exercises, postures, and breathing techniques was meant as a path to spiritual development. But today we know that yoga is great for all aspects of health, whether mental, physical, or spiritual.

There are several branches of yoga, although Raja and Hatha are the ones used most often in the United States. Through the use of postures, deep breathing, and progressive relaxation, yoga works to restore the *prana*, the life energy or vital force that flows through every living thing. Special yoga poses or postures (called *asanas*) help loosen and tone the muscles, relieve tension, increase flexibility, improve circulation, and ease the body into a state of relaxation. The breathing exercises (called *pranayama*) are designed to help restore the prana and keep it moving freely throughout the body, while expanding the capacity of the lungs, oxygenating the body, and slowing the breathing, heart rate, blood pressure, and metabolism. The progressive relaxation exercises help ease muscle tension, relieve stress, balance the nervous system, improve immune function, and make you feel like you just woke up from a deep, refreshing sleep. Ah, what could be more delicious!

AN ALL-AROUND ANTIDOTE TO PMS

Since PMS is made worse by stress, nervous tension, and emotional upsets, the relaxing, calming, and restorative effects of yoga may do much to ease your symptoms. But don't wait until you're in the middle of your next PMS-induced fit of anxiety to try yoga. A complex system of mental and physical training, yoga is referred to as a "discipline" for a good reason—it takes discipline and time to learn to apply its techniques correctly. And that means you can't just pick it up on the fly!

If you want to learn about yoga, be sure to study with a qualified yoga instructor, at least in the beginning. A good instructor will demonstrate the correct techniques, then watch to make sure you're assuming the positions correctly. If you just read a book or buy a videotape on yoga, you can end up stretching in the wrong way, which can strain the muscles and harm the body—exactly what you want to avoid! An instructor can also be indispensable as a guide through various relaxation exercises and a source of yoga-based spiritual enlightenment. Once you know what you're doing, you can do yoga on your own, just about any time, any place. But get some good face-to-face instruction initially.

YOGA EXERCISES FOR PMS RELIEF

While your instructor will certainly have his or her own favorite postures, I've outlined a few typical yoga exercises below that are known for promoting relaxation. Generally, the postures are assumed slowly and held for twenty seconds to two minutes, often in conjunction with deep breathing techniques. The deep breathing increases oxygenation of body tissues and aids in relaxation—both of which will help your body get the most out of each exercise. See your yoga instructor for detailed instructions on how to perform the following exercises.

Deep Breathing

Deep breathing fully oxygenates the body and increases relaxation. If you're like most people, you're a "chest breather." You breathe shallowly and don't fully expand your lungs, so your body is rarely oxygenated fully. And when you're stressed, your breathing gets even more shallow and rapid than usual. Luckily, this is easily remedied. Just by taking some deep, full breaths, you can set your body on the road to relaxation.

To learn to become a "lung breather" rather than a "chest breather," try the following:

1. Lie on your back, with knees bent, feet flat on the floor, and arms lying loosely by your sides.
2. Put your hands over your diaphragm, just underneath your sternum.
3. To the count of five, slowly and deeply inhale, inflating your diaphragm and using it to push your hands toward the ceiling. The rest of your body should remain completely relaxed as you do this.
4. Hold for a count of five, then contract your diaphragm and slowly push the air out, expelling every bit of the old, stale air. This way you'll be able to release any last little bit of air.
5. Repeat several times, completely filling and emptying your lungs each time.

Knee to Chest

This posture increases flexibility of the lower back, hip, and buttocks.

1. Lie on your back with your legs together and extended, with your arms at your sides.
2. As you slowly inhale, bend your right leg, grasp it with both hands just below the knee and bring it toward your chest, pulling it as far as it will go. (Try to keep your hips and rear end flat on the mat.)
3. Hold your bent leg at its maximum position for a count of five, while your other leg remains straight and in contact with the floor.
4. Slowly exhale as you release your leg and allow your body to return to its original position.
5. Repeat with the other leg. Do this exercise five times on each side.

Body Twist

The body twist increases the flexibility of the neck, chest, spine, and hip.

1. This is a more advanced version of the Knee-To-Chest exercise. Lie flat on your back with your legs together and extended, with your arms at your sides.
2. Bend your right leg, use both hands to clasp it just below the knee, and pull it gently toward your chest.
3. Then, using your left hand, pull your right knee across your body toward the floor beneath the left side of your hip.
4. At the same time, stretch your right arm out, letting it rest on the floor at a right angle to your body. As you press your knee toward the left, press your right shoulder blade to the floor on the right.

5. Turn your head to the right, toward your extended arm. Take a deep breath, exhale, and hold this position for a count of ten.
6. Slowly release and return to your original position.
7. Repeat using your right hand on your left knee, with your left arm extended to the side and your head turned toward the left.

The Pretzel

This posture increases the flexibility of the inner thigh and hip.

1. Lie on your back, with your knees bent and your arms relaxed at your sides.
2. Keeping your knees bent, cross your left ankle over your right thigh, just above your right knee. Your left foot should just clear your right thigh, and your left knee should point straight to the left.
3. As you slowly inhale, grab hold of the back of your right thigh with both hands and slowly pull it toward you without uncrossing your legs.
4. Hold for at least five seconds at your maximum position.
5. Slowly exhale as you release, and return to starting position.
6. Repeat with right ankle crossing your left thigh.

The Cat

The cat increases spinal flexibility.

1. Assume a "hands and knees" position as if you were a cat, weight distributed evenly between your palms and your knees, and fingers pointing straight ahead.
2. As you slowly inhale, pull your stomach muscles tight and curve your back toward the ceiling, like a cat that's arching

its back. Tuck your chin in toward your chest to complete the "cat-like" pose and hold for five counts.

3. Then, relax your spine and bring your head back to its normal position as you slowly exhale.

4. Continue exhaling as you reverse the arch of your spine, pulling your head back toward your upper back and swaying your back until it looks something like a shallow bowl. (Just sway a little: swaying a lot tends to crunch the vertebrae together.)

5. Begin inhaling again as your head, neck, and spine move back to starting position.

6. Continue inhaling as you repeat the exercise, first arching like a cat, then exhaling as you pull the head, neck, and spine backward. Do this exercise slowly and easily; never rush.

The Snake

This posture increases the flexibility of the chest, stomach, and back muscles and strengthens the arms and upper body.

1. Lie facedown on a mat with elbows bent and palms pressed flat against the mat on either side of the neck. Fingers should be parallel to the sides of your neck.

2. As you slowly inhale, press the palms into the mat and use the lower arms to help you slowly raise your head and upper chest until they are completely off the floor. At the maximum position, your eyes should be about horizon level; don't throw your head backward.

3. Then gradually straighten your arms as you push your head, chest, and torso as far off the mat as they'll go. Keep the pelvis flat on the floor, with legs extended. Again, keep the eyes at horizon level; head and neck should be perpendicular to the floor.

4. Hold for a count of five.
5. Exhale slowly as you bend your arms and gradually ease your torso, head, and neck back down to the original starting position on the mat.
6. Repeat five times.

The Child's Pose

The child's pose increases spinal flexibility and aids in relaxation. This is a great one to do at the end of your session to ease your body into a totally relaxed state.

1. Tuck your legs underneath you as you sit on a mat, with your heels directly underneath your rear end and your knees pointing forward.
2. Pull your knees apart about ten inches while keeping toes together, forming a "V" with your thighs that meets at your toes.
3. Roll your upper body forward to the floor, with your arms extended loosely in front of you. Your forehead should touch the floor if possible. (Separate your knees even more, if necessary, to get your forehead to touch the floor, but keep your rear end in contact with your heels.)
4. Relax in this position for a count of twenty, or as long as you like.
5. Slowly roll up to a sitting position.

TO FIND A QUALIFIED YOGA INSTRUCTOR . . .

To learn more about yoga and find out how to choose a good yoga instructor, contact the American Yoga Association, P.O. Box 19986, Sarasota, FL 34276; phone: (800) 226-5859; website: www .americanyogaassociation.org, then click on "Yoga Teachers."

17

DLPA

There's a surprisingly helpful remedy for PMS sitting on the shelves of many vitamin stores. It's an amino acid called DLPA, which stands for *dl-phenylalanine*. DLPA was first introduced to the public back in the 1980s as a way to combat chronic pain and depression. What makes it unique is that it is completely unlike pain pills, which are designed to reduce inflammation and/or suppress the release of certain "pain chemicals" in the body. It also works its magic in a very different way from the antidepressants that so many people take on a daily basis. That's because DLPA doesn't directly attack either pain or depression. Instead, it acts as a kind of "bodyguard" for certain hormones that act as natural painkillers and mood elevators. So instead of just barging in and forcibly rearranging your internal chemistry like drugs do, DLPA takes a gentler approach. It lends a hand to your very own hormones and encourages your body to heal itself. As a result, your mood improves and you experience less pain, but don't have to deal with the nasty side effects of painkilling or antidepressant drugs.

PROTECTING THE PAINKILLERS

To understand how DLPA works, you'll need to know something about endorphins, your body's natural antidotes to pain and depression. The word *endorphin* is a combination of the words "endogenous" and "morphine," which means "the morphine within"—and morphine, of course, is the strongest painkiller in existence. Happily, it's true; your endorphins do function as your own personal brand of morphine.

Why do you need your own personal painkillers? Because you, like everybody else, have a certain amount of "background" pain that's always present and that you don't really need to know about. While you *do* need to know about certain kinds of pain for survival's sake (like when you accidentally touch a hot stove or you hit your thumb with a hammer), you *don't* really need to be reminded about the gash in your leg that's been healing for a week, the bruise you got when you ran into the sharp corner of a table, or the general aches and pains that seem to hang around for no discernible reason. These pain messages aren't telling you that you're endangering your body. They're just pointless aggravation that can end up making your life miserable.

The job of the endorphins is to suppress these kinds of meaningless pain messages. They are the "feel good" hormones that are responsible for the "runner's high," which kicks in at a certain point to block the pain of running and help the runner feel great. But sometimes the endorphins fall down on the job and the unnecessary kind of pain messages start to break through. Why does this happen? Either your body doesn't make enough endorphins, or those that it does make die off too quickly. Either way, you end up with too few endorphins and too much meaningless pain.

PMS AND THE ENDORPHINS

What does all of this have to do with PMS? One of the theories of the origins of PMS is that it's due to a withdrawal from our internal narcotic, the endorphins. Interestingly enough, the description of PMS symptoms given by some women (anxiety, restlessness, abdominal cramps, nausea) sounds like the symptoms of narcotic withdrawal. Some researchers theorize that the endorphin levels in some women plummet during the week before menstruation, bringing on PMS symptoms. Or perhaps these women just become less sensitive to the painkilling, antidepressive effects of the endorphins during the premenstrual phase. Either way, the endorphin "shield" against pain and depression seems to weaken right around the week before the menstrual period, at least in certain women.

If you could find a way to raise your endorphin levels, especially at this time, you might be able to ward off PMS and a host of other ailments related to pain and depression. Unfortunately, you can't just take a pill or get a shot of endorphins. The body doesn't work that way. And currently, there's no effective way of stimulating the body to make more endorphins, either. There's only one way to pump up your endorphin supply: you've got to *protect* the endorphins that you already have from destruction. Then your endorphin supply can slowly build up. You can do this by taking a simple amino acid called *phenylalanine*.

A LITTLE BACKGROUND ON THE "ENDORPHIN SHIELD"

Like other amino acids, phenylalanine comes in two forms: D and L. These two forms are like your right and left hands, identical but reversed, forming mirror images of each other. You can find the two forms separately, labeled DPA and LPA, or together as the 50/50 mix known as DLPA, the form that's most effective and is recommended for daily use.

How powerful is DLPA? Well, the relief offered by typical pain pills is often measured in terms of hours: four hours, six hours, or perhaps twelve. That's why you have to keep taking pain pills throughout the day. But the relief provided by DLPA lasts for days, often four days or more.

DLPA also helps lift certain forms of depression. I'm not referring to the kind of depression that strikes when we suffer a personal loss or tragedy. That's called *reactive depression*, and it's an understandable response that will fade with time. Instead, DLPA helps work on the kind of depression that seems to strike for no reason, a much more paralyzing condition that is probably due to faulty biochemistry. In various studies, DLPA has eased this kind of depression every bit as well as standard medicines and, in some cases, has proved to be even more effective.

A PAIN RELIEVER WITHOUT SIDE EFFECTS

And there's more good news. While you can develop a tolerance or even an addiction to aspirin, narcotics, and other pain-relieving medications, you can't develop a tolerance or addiction to DLPA. While you can suffer quite serious side effects from standard pain and depression medicines, DLPA has no side effects. And while pain pills can be dangerous or even life-threatening when overused, DLPA is on the U.S. government's GRAS (Generally Recognized As Safe) list.

HOW MUCH DO YOU NEED?

While there are no hard-and-fast rules regarding DLPA dosages, here are some general guidelines:

- If you weigh at least 110 pounds, start by taking 750 mg of DLPA a day—half with breakfast and half with lunch. If you weigh less, take a little less.
- Give DLPA a chance to work. Remember, it's not a pain pill like aspirin or Tylenol that starts working right away. It's a longer, more involved process.
- Although DLPA begins protecting your endorphins soon after you take it, you'll need to allow time for the endorphins to accu-

mulate in your body before they can effectively combat pain and depression. It may take up to two weeks before you feel any relief, so start taking DLPA at least ten days before your PMS symptoms usually appear. If you try to take it as an on-the-spot pain reliever, you'll be disappointed.

BEFORE YOU TAKE DLPA . . .

If you'd like to try DLPA, consult with your physician first. DLPA should not be used by pregnant or lactating women, those on phenylalanine-restricted diets, or those who have the genetic disease phenylketonuria (PKU), a condition in which phenylalanine cannot be metabolized properly.

18

Homeopathy

Homeopathy is a popular healing art based on the idea that taking a tiny dose of whatever's ailing you can be the best treatment for that same disease. The name "homeopathy" literally means "similar suffering," and the way it works can be compared to that of a vaccine. With a polio vaccine, for example, you are injected with a very tiny amount of the polio virus—not enough to make you sick, just enough to stimulate the production of polio antibodies within your body. Then, should you ever be exposed to the "real" polio virus, you'll already have the antibodies on board that can fight it off. In short, your immune system has become "primed" because of its exposure to the enemy. Homeopathy works in a similar way. By taking a little bit of whatever would cause your ailment in a healthy person, you can shift your own natural defenses into high gear and affect a "cure." But unlike a vaccination, the homeopathic medicines are taken when you're already in the throes of an ailment. In other words, homeopathic remedies are used to cure rather than prevent disease.

THE WEAKER IT IS, THE STRONGER IT IS . . .

A basic tenet of homeopathy is the more diluted the remedy is, the stronger it becomes. Therefore, each homeopathic medicine or remedy contains an extremely small dose of its active ingredient. For example, a typical homeopathic remedy is made by combining one drop of the active ingredient with nine drops of a water/alcohol solution (or similar diluting substance). After thoroughly mixing the ten drops, one drop of this "new" solution is removed and mixed with nine drops of yet another diluting solution. So the end result may be one hundred times more dilute than the original active ingredient—making it almost undetectable. But according to homeopaths, this new solution is much stronger now than it was at the beginning of the diluting process.

HOMEOPATHY TREATS YOUR "ESSENCE"

The homeopathic physician believes that physical symptoms (like PMS) are the result of certain physical, mental, and emotional upsets to your very essence—the "inner you." So rather than trying to treat the outer symptoms, he or she will attempt to reach inside and calm the turmoil that caused the problem in the first place. In order to do this, the homeopathic physician will need to get information about the "inner you" to determine the nature of your essence. For example, he or she may ask you about your likes and dislikes, your family life, your stressors, the length and quality of your sleep, your weather preferences, etc. Then you'll need to give a detailed account of your symptoms, when they strike, what you're usually doing at the time, how long they last, and so on. (Your PMS diary will help you answer these questions more accurately and completely.) Once the homeopathic physician has built a "subjective data base" on your inner self, he or she can form an idea of your essence and decide on the kind of remedy that would suit you best.

THE HOMEOPATHIC PRESCRIPTION FOR PMS

You'll need to see a qualified homeopathic physician to find out which remedies are best for you and to get complete instructions on how much to take and when. But for your own information, I've listed some of the remedies typically prescribed for PMS, with the common name listed first and the proper name in parentheses.

- **Calc Carb** (*Calcarea carboica-ostrearum*)—For tender, swollen breasts prior to menstrual period.
- **Kali Phos** (*Kali phosphoricum*)—For anxiety, late or scanty periods, or loss of periods accompanied by severe depression.
- **Lachesis** (*Lachesis*)—For extremes of mood, including anxiety, depression, sorrow, vexation, and/or jealousy. All complaints are worse after sleep, warm baths, or hot drinks. For hot flashes, perspiration, sleeplessness, heart palpitations, and back pain that radiates to the hips and legs. Symptoms are greatly relieved once the menstrual period starts.
- **Nat Mur** (*Natrum muriaticum*)—For depression, irritability, changeable moods (i.e., tears to laughter), throbbing headache, vaginal dryness, severe lower-back pain, and great weariness upon arising. Also for salt cravings and abdominal bloating.
- **Pulsatilla** (*Pulsatilla*)—For delayed periods, abdominal distension, difficulty falling asleep, and restless sleep. Also for moodiness and shooting pains in the neck and upper back.
- **Sepia** (*Sepia*)—For severe headache, hot flashes, indigestion, nausea, vomiting, irregular periods, and lower-back pain that is worse when standing. Also, for unrefreshing sleep, bloated abdomen, depres-

sion, indifference to family accompanied by dread of being alone, and the sensation that the pelvic contents are about to fall out.

There are also remedies specifically geared to migraines, including:

- **Cimicifuga** (*Cimicifuga racemosa*)—For a migraine that seems to be pressing outward from the inside of the skull and appears after long-term worry or study.
- **Scutellaria** (*Scutellaria*)—For a migraine that produces a dull pain in the front of the head, reddening of the face, and restlessness.

A WORD OF WARNING

When you take homeopathic remedies, you may end up feeling *worse* instead of better, at least at first. That's because the remedy is designed to get your immune system to gear up by thinking you're a "little bit" sick. This method is aimed at attacking the inner, essential problem that's affecting you on the physical, mental, or emotional level. And that can take some time. So don't expect to take a homeopathic remedy and—voila!—your PMS is gone. Give it some time to "take" before you decide that it's all hokum. And don't try to self-treat. Homeopathy is too complex for the amateur. Your best bet is to find a trained homeopathic physician and give it at least six months before deciding whether or not homeopathy works for you.

TO FIND A QUALIFIED HOMEOPATHIC PHYSICIAN . . .

You can get a list of trained homeopathic physicians by contacting the National Center for Homeopathy, 801 N. Fairfax St., Suite 306, Alexandria, VA 22314; phone: (703) 548-7790, website: www .homeopathic.org.

19

Aromatherapy

Ever since I was a little girl, I've noticed that certain smells have the ability to transport me to a specific time and place or call up strong emotions, all in an instant. One whiff of lighter fluid, for example, and I can remember exactly how it felt to be four years old, standing on a chair in our kitchen, and watching my daddy refill his shiny silver cigarette lighter. The smell of cherry tobacco immediately gives me a warm and fuzzy feeling because my best friend's father used to smoke a pipe with that kind of tobacco, and I always liked being in her house. Clearly, scents are stimulating to our brains and can affect our moods, stress levels, metabolism, and even libido. This, then, is the basis of the healing art of aromatherapy.

THE ESSENCE OF ESSENTIAL OILS

The special aromas used in aromatherapy come from concentrated extracts taken from different flowers, herbs, grasses, shrubs, and trees. These extracts are called *essential oils* and have been used as healing agents for body and mind for centuries. In theory, each essential oil exerts a particular effect on the mind and/or body, and the oils are often classified according to these effects. For example, some affect the physical body: they may have antiseptic properties, help ease bronchial congestion, increase the circulation, heal wounds, regulate the blood pressure, or ease muscle spasms. Others are used primarily for their psychological effects: they can calm, sedate, excite, stimulate, or even bring about a sense of euphoria.

True essential oils are extracted from the roots, flowers, leaves, or stalks of organically grown plants or trees via steam distillation, solvent extraction, or peel pressure. The resulting scent is very concentrated and aromatic and loaded with organic compounds that have positive effects on the hypothalamus, a part of the brain that regulates mood. The oils are made up of tiny molecules that are easy to absorb through the bronchial passages and skin into the bloodstream. Aromatherapists insist that synthetic "knock-offs" of essential oils (sometimes marketed under the catchall term *aromacology*) do not produce the same therapeutic effects, since they lack the organic compounds.

Although the essential oils are normally sold in their undiluted state, they're much too strong to apply directly to the skin. If you're planning to use them for a massage, you'll need to purchase a *carrier oil*, such as sweet almond, apricot kernel, or sunflower oil, to use for dilution purposes. Normally, 20 ml of carrier oil is used to dilute ten drops of essential oil. (Reduce to five drops of essential oil if your skin is sensitive.)

USING ESSENTIAL OILS

The healing aromas of essential oils can be administered in several ways:

- Add a few drops of essential oil to a pot of boiling water, then remove from heat and let it cool for two to three minutes. Drape a towel over both your head and the pot to keep the steam from escaping and gently inhale. (Note: To avoid steam burns, make sure the contents of the pot have cooled sufficiently before inhaling.)

- Use a humidifier, and add a few drops of essential oil to its water supply.
- Try a diffuser, a nebulizer, or a vaporizer to fill the entire room with aroma. (These accessories are available from aromatherapy manufacturers.)
- During a massage, use a carrier oil mixed with a few drops of essential oil.
- Add some essential oil to your bathwater.
- Certain oils (e.g., jasmine) can be added to a hot cup of tea and sipped.

AROMAS FOR PMS

The essential oils that are typically prescribed by aromatherapists for general PMS symptoms include:

- Chamomile (*Matricaria chamomilla*)
- Clary sage (*Salvia sclarea*)
- Geranium (*Pelargonium odorantissimum*)
- Lavender (*Lavandula officinalis*)
- Melissa (*Melissa officinalis*)
- Rose (*Rosa centifolia*)
- Rosemary (*Rosmarinus officinalis*)
- Sandalwood (*Santalum album*)

For anxiety or nervous tension, try:

- Benzoin (*Styrax benzoin*)
- Bergamot (*Monarda didyma*)
- Camphor (*Cinnamomum camphora*)
- Chamomile (*Matricaria chamomilla*)
- Cypress (*Cupressus sempervirens*)

- Lavender (*Lavandula officinalis*)
- Melissa (*Melissa officinalis*)
- Patchouli (*Pogostemon patchouli*)

For breast tenderness or water retention:

- Geranium (*Pelargonium odorantissimum*)
- Juniper (*Juniperus communis*)
- Lavender (*Lavandula officinalis*)

For depression:

- Basil (*Ocimum basilicum*)
- Bergamot (*Monarda didyma*)
- Camphor (*Cinnamomum camphora*)
- Geranium (*Pelargonium odorantissimum*)
- Jasmine (*Jasminum officinale*)
- Lavender (*Lavandula officinalis*)
- Neroli (*Citrus aurantium*)

For headaches (migraine or otherwise):

- Basil (*Ocimum basilicum*)
- Chamomile (*Matricaria chamomilla*)
- Eucalyptus (*Eucalyptus globules*)
- Lavender (*Lavandula officinalis*)
- Marjoram (*Origanum marjorana*)
- Melissa (*Melissa officinalis*)
- Rose (*Rosa centifolia*)
- Rosemary (*Rosmarinus officinalis*)

For insomnia:

- Basil (*Ocimum basilicum*)
- Chamomile (*Matricaria chamomilla*)
- Juniper (*Juniperus communis*)
- Marjoram (*Origanum marjorana*)
- Rose (*Rosa centifolia*)

- Sandalwood (*Santalum album*)
- Ylang-ylang (*Cananga odorata*)

For irregular periods:

- Basil (*Ocimum basilicum*)
- Clary sage (*Salvia sclarea*)
- Jasmine (*Jasminum officinale*)
- Juniper (*Juniperus communis*)
- Lavender (*Lavandula officinalis*)
- Melissa (*Melissa officinalis*)
- Rose (*Rosa centifolia*)

For fatigue:

- Basil (*Ocimum basilicum*)
- Geranium (*Pelargonium odorantissimum*)
- Marjoram (*Origanum marjorana*)
- Rosemary (*Rosmarinus officinalis*)

TO FIND A QUALIFIED AROMATHERAPIST . . .

It's best to begin aromatherapy under the guidance of a qualified aromatherapist who can help you find your way through the maze of aromas and aroma delivery systems. Once you know what you're doing, you can continue on your own. To find a qualified aromatherapist, contact the National Association for Holistic Aromatherapy (NAHA), P.O. Box 17622, Boulder, CO 80308; phone: (303) 258-3791; website: www.naha.org.

20

Massage

Just about everybody likes a good massage, undoubtedly one of the oldest healing arts in existence. The "laying on of hands" can be soothing, comforting, stimulating, and relaxing—all at once!—in ways that simply can't be reproduced by any artificial means. And when you're uptight, stressed out, irritable, depressed, or feeling like you want to scream (in short, when you're suffering from PMS), a good massage can be exactly what you need. But relaxation and stress relief aren't the only benefits of a good rubdown. Other terrific "side effects" include improved circulation, enhanced nervous-system function, stimulation of a sluggish metabolism, decreased blood pressure, increased levels of endorphins, improved sleep, and relief from pain. If you could market the effects of massage in pill form, you'd become a multimillionaire!

WHICH KIND OF MASSAGE WORKS BEST FOR PMS?

The world of massage includes a host of methods, ranging from the kind that can send you into dreamland to the kind that can make you feel like you've gone a couple of rounds in the boxing ring. The kind that's most often performed, and the kind that may be most helpful for easing PMS, is *Swedish massage*, also known as *effleurage*. The skin and muscles are gently kneaded and stroked, with extra pressure exerted on tight, knotted muscles to break up tension and encourage relaxation. Swedish massage is great for relieving the stress and tension that can build up during the PMS phase. It also helps to stimulate the movement of body fluids, thus increasing the amount of nutrients and oxygen delivered to the cells, while speeding the removal of toxins.

To work on specific areas that hold tension, you may want to try *shiatsu* (another name for acupressure), which involves pressure placed on various "acupoints" on the body to break up and release energy blockages. The pressure is not necessarily exerted where you feel pain; instead the acupoints are stimulated to release blocked energy in one particular area, which can speed the healing of areas "downstream" from that point. For example, if you've got cramps in your lower back, the massage therapist may press on a point further up your spine to release a blockage and allow your lower-back pain to heal. (For a more complete explanation, see Chapter 21.)

For PMS, Swedish massage and shiatsu are probably your best bets since they emphasize relaxation and the release of tension using pain-free methods. More intense massage methods such as myofascial release, deep tissue massage, and Rolfing are probably too stimulating and painful during this time. The main thing to remember about a massage designed to relieve PMS symptoms is that it should feel good. If it doesn't, speak up! Your massage therapist should welcome your feedback and be willing to adjust the pressure and/or technique immediately until you feel comfortable.

GETTING THE MOST OUT OF YOUR MASSAGE

What you do before, during, and after the massage can either maximize its relaxing effects or practically negate the whole experience. To make the most of your massage, consider the following tips:

- Schedule your massage for the time of the month when your PMS symptoms are typically at their worst. If possible, try to make the appointment during a less-busy time in your schedule, like a weekend, a day off, or later in the evening. That way, you won't have to dash in from work, shopping, or some other high-energy task or, worse yet, dash off immediately afterward.
- Take a warm bath or shower in advance to loosen up your muscles and get yourself into a relaxation mode.
- Tell the therapist about any symptoms you're currently experiencing. Also, let him or her know what massage techniques you like and don't like (for example, no intense pressure on the arch of my foot!). If you're not sure, ask about what he or she usually does and be clear about what does and does not appeal to you.
- Then, once you're into the massage, relax completely. Let it all go as you drift into a dreamy state.
- Be sure to give feedback during the massage: what hurts, what feels good, where you think you'd like more or less pressure, and so on.
- Then, when the massage is finished, take a few minutes to lie on the table and continue relaxing. Don't immediately leap up, get dressed and race back into your life! If you're at home, take a nap or just lie down for a while. If you're at a spa, take a whirlpool bath or relax in the sauna. Then slowly get dressed and ease back into the real world.
- Finally, drink plenty of water after your massage to help your body flush out circulating toxins. Massage increases the circulation of the lymph, which contains the body's waste material, and drinking extra water helps flush wastes away more quickly.

TO FIND A GOOD MASSAGE THERAPIST . . .

To find a certified massage therapist, get a referral from the American Massage Therapy Association, 820 Davis Street, Suite 100, Evanston,

IL 60201; phone: (847) 864-0123; website: www.amtamassage.org or The National Certification Board for Therapeutic Massage and Bodywork, 8301 Greensboro Drive, Suite 300, McLean, VA 22102; phone: (800) 296-0664; website: www.ncbtmb.com.

21

Acupuncture and Acupressure

For thousands of years, traditional Chinese medicine has espoused the use of acupressure and acupuncture as effective methods of easing pain and treating a myriad of ailments. Both are based on the idea that the body is filled with *qi* (pronounced "chee"), the "life energy," which is distributed throughout the body through a network of invisible channels called *meridians*. The meridians snake their way through the body like subterranean energy rivers, and occasionally rise to the surface, where they flow just underneath the skin. The points at which the meridians near the surface are called *acupoints*.

According to the theory of Traditional Chinese Medicine, when the qi is flowing freely, all is well within the body and good health reigns. But if the flow of qi slows or becomes blocked, a stagnation of energy occurs which is thought to be the root of all disease.

UNBLOCKING THE ENERGY

You can think of a blockage of qi within a meridian as something like a dirt clod in one of your main sprinkler lines. As long as the dirt clod remains, your sprinkler line will be unable to deliver water to all of the sprinkler heads that it serves. As a result, the plants that depend on water from those sprinkler heads will dry up and wither away. Similarly, when the flow of qi slows down or is blocked off, the parts of the body serviced by that particular meridian will suffer. If the blockage happens to occur in the meridians that serve the female organs, PMS can be the unhappy result.

To clear a block in your sprinkler line, you may have to blow it out with a high-pressure stream of water or even dig up the line, cut off the offending part, and replace it. But that's not possible with blocked qi. Instead, you simply stimulate certain *acupoints*, to help break up the blockages and get the qi moving again. When the stimulation involves the application of manual pressure, it's called *acupressure* (or *shiatsu* in Japanese). When it involves the insertion of very fine needles, it's called *acupuncture*. Either method is believed to help restore the flow of qi, thus allowing the body to heal itself.

ACUPRESSURE FOR PMS

Acupressure is performed by acupressurists, acupuncturists, most massage therapists, and some physical therapists. You can even perform it on yourself once you've learned the basics. Blockages in the qi are broken up by applying pressure to various acupoints using the fingers, thumbs, elbows, wooden rollers, balls, pointers, or other tools. Acupressure should always be performed smoothly and gradually, with a firm, steady force. Enough pressure should be exerted to cause a "good hurt" without producing real pain. Often the practitioner will make a circular motion while exerting the pressure to help diffuse the force and prevent tissue damage. Rolling motions, vibrating, the kneading of the tissues, or rotating pressure can also be used.

Besides freeing the qi and recharging energy levels, these techniques can help stimulate circulation and increase relaxation. When applied to the acupoints governing the female organs, acupressure may help ease lower-back pain, menstrual cramps, fluid retention, and muscle tension. It's also used to counteract stress, fatigue, headaches, migraines, depression, anxiety, and insomnia.

During an acupressure session, make sure you maintain deep, rhythmic breathing and try to relax and give into the pressure. Don't hold your breath, or you'll contribute to a buildup of lactic acid that can cause further pain.

ACUPUNCTURE FOR PMS

According to the theory of acupuncture, the acupoints are connected to nerve receptors, and when very fine stainless-steel needles are inserted into these points, nerve cells are stimulated and pain decreases. This may be due to the release of endorphins, the body's naural painkillers. Or it may have to do with the Gate Theory of Pain, which suggests that the nerve pathways have "gates" that open and close either to let pain messages through or block them. Acupuncture may close the "gates," so that fewer pain messages reach the brain; therefore, you feel less pain. The truth is, no one is quite sure just how acupuncture works, but studies done on this ancient healing art have shown that it does stimulate both the immune and circulatory systems.

When you first visit an acupuncturist, you may be surprised at the length and the depth of the interview that you'll go through. A basic tenet of Traditional Chinese Medicine is the assessment of your condition using the "Four Examinations"—the first of which is *asking* (about your history, symptoms, the location and intensity of your pain, your diet, sleeping habits, bowel habits, and emotional state.) Next comes *observing*, when the acupuncturist examines your eyes, skin, tongue, and fingernails. Then there's the *listening* phase, during which he or she will listen to your speaking voice, bowel sounds, and breathing. Finally, there's the *touching* portion, when various parts of your body will be touched to detect areas of tenderness and/or emptiness, as well as changes in skin temperature. Your pulse will be taken in twelve different areas to check the rhythm and strength of all twelve meridians. The idea is to find out where the imbalance exists within your body. This is particularly important in PMS, which involves a wide range of symptoms that are almost certainly related to internal imbalances.

HOW ACUPUNCTURE IS DONE

Your acupuncture session will most likely involve one or more of the following treatments:

• **Inserting acupuncture needles**—Very thin, hair-like acupuncture needles are eased into the designated acupoints to a depth of between ⅛ and 1 inch. Usually between six and twelve needles are used and they're left in place for a few seconds, several minutes, or even as long as an hour. Sometimes the acupuncturist will insert the needles, then attach them to a machine via tiny wires that deliver a low-grade dose of electricity. The electricity makes the needles vibrate slightly, offering greater stimulation to the nerves, which is supposed to increase the effectiveness of the treatment. If the vibration becomes uncomfortable or annoying, the intensity of the current can be lowered.

• **Moxibustion (burning of herbs)**—An herb called moxa is burned over the acupuncture points to stimulate them. A small amount of the herb is placed on a piece of cardboard, which is then placed directly on the acupoint. As the herb slowly burns, the acupoint is stimulated by the heat, but if the heat becomes uncomfortable, the moxa is immediately removed.

• **Cupping**—When little glass cups are warmed and put upside-down over the acupuncture points, they create a vacuum effect that draws qi and blood toward them, stimulating the area.

Sometimes it takes five or six sessions before acupuncture brings results, so if you decide to try it, be sure to give it a good run before evaluating its effectiveness. For best results, get regular treatments a couple of times a week for at least two months. Once pain relief is achieved, you may want to reduce your treatments to once a week or once every other week.

TO FIND A QUALIFIED PRACTITIONER . . .

Although you can learn to perform acupressure on yourself, acupuncture should always be done by a professional, since it's an invasive treatment. You can find a good practitioner of either acupuncture or acupressure by contacting the National Certification Commission for Acupuncture and Oriental Medicine (NCCAOM), 11 Canal Center Plaza, Suite 330, Alexandria, VA 22314; phone: (703) 548-9004; website: www.nccaom.org.

Since acupressure (shiatsu) is practiced by a great many massage therapists, you can find a practitioner skilled in this healing art by contacting the American Massage Therapy Association, 820 Davis Street, Suite 100, Evanston, IL 60201; phone: (847) 864-0123; E-mail: info@inet.amtamassage.org; website: www.amtamassage.org. Or consult your doctor, chiropractor and/or physical therapist for referrals.

22

Reflexology

Can a foot massage possibly relieve your PMS? According to enthu-siasts of reflexology, the answer is a resounding "yes"! An ancient heal-ing art dating back to the Egyptians in 2300 B.C., reflexology involves gentle to strong pressure exerted on specific points found on the feet, hands, or outer ears to break up energy blockages and restore the free flow of qi, the body's life force. Proponents of reflexology say it's an excellent way to relieve tension, improve circulation, stimulate the nerves, normalize both nerve and gland function, and restore balance to the body. And, although pressing points on your feet, hands, or ears to restore balance to your body may sound far-fetched, there is some scientific proof of its effectiveness. A whopping three hundred studies performed in China, involving a total of eighteen thousand individual cases and sixty-four different illnesses, showed that reflex-ology had a positive effect on patients 95 percent of the time. Even more to the point, a 1991 study performed at UCLA found that women who received weekly reflexology treatments for PMS reduced their symptoms by 62 percent!

The popularity of reflexology has grown in recent years and its healing capabilities have been officially recognized by medical establishments and/or business corporations in several different countries throughout the world. In the United Kingdom, Australia, and New Zealand, reflexology is widely used in pain clinics, cancer centers, and neonatal clinics. In Denmark and Japan, several large corporations include benefits for reflexology treatments in their health plans, since studies have shown that employees who see reflexologists take fewer sick days. And in the United States, reflexology is finally beginning to shed its reputation as acupressure's "kid sister."

HOW DOES REFLEXOLOGY WORK?

Reflexology is based on the idea that all the organs, glands, and systems of the body are linked through the nerves to *reflex points* on the soles of the feet. The hands and ears also have certain points that correspond to various body parts. Using special thumb, finger, and hand techniques to manipulate these points, the reflexologist promotes relaxation and enhances wellness, especially in the corresponding area of the body.

A map of the reflex points that correspond to different areas of the body can be constructed on the soles of the feet. Imagine that the body is divided into ten reflex-energy "zones" that run lengthwise from the top of the head through the tip of each toe and also down the arm through the end of each finger. When looking at the soles of the feet, these ten reflex-energy zones also run straight down from the tip of each toe to the heel. So when looking at both soles of the feet, there are ten lengthwise sections.

Then the sole is divided horizontally into four zones. Each of these zones corresponds to a major area of the body: for example, the heel corresponds to the lower abdominal and pelvic regions, the arch of the foot to the upper and mid-abdominal regions, the ball of the foot to the chest region, and the toes to the head and neck region. The top and the side of the foot also have a few reflex points. So no matter what part of your body hurts or is suffering from an imbalance, there's a corresponding point on your foot that can be stimulated by the reflexologist. Yet reflexology is not just aimed at "fixing" a particular part of your body. It's meant to improve the function of *all* of your organs, glands, and body systems through the restoration of balance.

WHAT GOES ON IN A REFLEXOLOGY SESSION

When the reflexologist treats you for PMS, she'll stimulate all of the major reflex areas on your foot, and then will pay particular attention to the areas that correlate with your pelvis and female organs. The area of the foot dedicated to the pelvis is the heel, while the inside of the upper arch governs the adrenal glands. The reflex point for the uterus is found on the inside of the ankle just above the heel. A corresponding point on the outside of the ankle rules the ovaries, and an imaginary band stretching between these two points governs the fallopian tubes. The reflexologist will stimulate all of these areas one by one, using special thumb and finger techniques that may feel like someone is drawing very definite lines with a fingernail on the sole of your foot and up and down the insides of your toes. (It's not a fingernail; it's the side of the reflexologist's thumb bone. But it does exert a well-defined, almost sharp pressure.)

As the reflexologist works, he or she will be able to feel an imbalance in your body in the form of a granular or crystalline deposit underneath the surface of a reflex point. You'll be able to feel it as a tenderness that makes you go "ouch!" when he or she starts pressing on it. But the more pain you feel, the more imbalanced your body is in that area—and that means you really need the stimulation there. So some pain is a "good hurt." And at the end of your treatment, you should find yourself as relaxed as if you'd had a full body massage.

TO FIND A QUALIFIED REFLEXOLOGIST . . .

Your best bet is to ask for a list of referrals from the Reflexology Association of America, 4012 Rainbow Blvd., Suite K, Box 585, Las Vegas, NV 89103-2059; phone: (702) 871-9522; website: www .reflexology-usa.org.

23

Positive Thinking

"I've got some positive thoughts for you," my friend Kelly told me. "I would positively like to poke my fingers in my husband's eyes every time he says 'It must be that time of the month'! I would positively like to rip my 'PMS genes' out of my body. And I would positively like to carry a stun gun and zap everybody who gets on my nerves during 'that time.'"

Of course, that wasn't quite the definition of "positive" I had in mind when I told Kelly that she might be able to decrease some of her PMS symptoms by thinking positively. Okay, then, I'll put it another way. Negative thinking, the kind we all *love* to indulge in now and then, can actually alter your body chemistry so that everything that already hurts feels even worse! Anger, frustration, and negative thinking all encourage the body to produce more stress hormones, particularly cortisol, and these can eat into your progesterone supply and cause hormone imbalances. Thus, you end up feeling even worse.

YOU ARE WHAT YOU THINK

Bear with me for just a moment while we take a peek at the science behind positive and negative thinking. It begins, oddly enough, with rocket ships. More specifically, with the rocket scientists who, in the late 1960s and early 1970s, astonished the world by making it possible for astronauts to walk on the moon. These guys really had it made: they were admired, applauded, well-paid, and racking up one incredible success after another. But they were also remarkably likely to suffer from what doctors called "sudden heart death." This was puzzling, because their cholesterol levels weren't any higher than average, they didn't smoke or drink more than average, and didn't have higher blood pressure than other groups. So why were these successful scientists so good at dying young?

Well, the truth of the matter was that along with the accolades and big paychecks came an extremely high likelihood of being fired. You see, our government kept a close eye on the space program budget, and every time we leapt ahead of the Russians by firing off another rocket, the government felt "safe" enough to fire another bunch of scientists. So, ironically, the more these men succeeded, the more likely they were to find themselves on unemployment. Not surprisingly, these scientists tended to have minds filled with fear, doubt, uncertainty, and other negative thoughts. They also felt helpless and hopeless. When doctors autopsied the unhappy men who died too young, they found that large portions of their hearts had been destroyed by the adrenaline, cortisol, and other powerful chemicals that the body pumps out when it's awash in negative feelings. In other words, their unhappy feelings had literally broken their hearts.

You can see the same thing in laboratory animals. If, for example, you inject large amounts of "stress chemicals" into lab animals, they will die from the same sort of heart damage that killed the scientists. Rabbits who are rotated between comfortable cages and uncomfortable, highly overcrowded cages, will die within six months from the stress and uncertainty. If you put an aggressive tree shrew in one cage and a submissive one in another, but let them see each other, the submissive shrew will die from fear in just a few weeks.

ACCENTUATE THE POSITIVE, ELIMINATE THE NEGATIVE

That's the bad news—now for some good. You've heard about place-bos, those "sugar pills" that contain no actual medicine but manage to make a lot of people feel better. In study after study, placebos have "cured" an incredible number and variety of diseases, from headaches to depression to chest pain. Why? Because they tap into the patients' positive thoughts. If the patients believe that the placebo is real med-icine and that it will really help, they tend to get better. That's because these positive thoughts actually rearrange body chemistry, lowering the production of adrenalin and other "stress chemicals," while increasing the production of endorphins and other "good" body chemicals. Doctors have been able to measure the positive changes in people brought about by placebos, and these changes prove that good thoughts really can enhance health and relieve stress.

Luckily, we don't have to wait until we take a placebo to start enjoy-ing the benefits of positive thinking. We can prescribe our own "placebos" just by thinking positive thoughts. Focus on the good things in your life. Think about fun, love, a good joke, where you want to go on your next vacation, and all the many successes you've achieved in life. Appreciate the beauty that surrounds you—the beau-tiful faces of those you love, your flower garden, a nearby park. Cre-ate visions of serenity in your mind—a quiet day on a warm deserted beach, a walk in a pine-scented forest, the mist of a beautiful foun-tain drifting over your face. Think about the wonder of nature or the majesty of God. Look for little things to be happy about in your life.

The partner to positive thinking is the "cancelling out" of negative thoughts. If you're mad at your husband, think about the many good times you've had together. Remember that magic moment when you realized he was "the one," and how great it felt. Think about the first time you held hands, or when he first told you that he loved you. If your boss is driving you crazy, think about how much fun you'll have this weekend, what you're going to do with your paycheck, or how cute your baby is. As my mother used to say, "Just let it go, like water off a duck's back."

THE BEST MEDICINE

There's no magic formula—just think good thoughts whenever possible. Remember: positive thinking is your very own always-available remedy for whatever ails you. Thinking positively will automatically reduce stress—and anything that cuts back on stress is bound to make you feel better.

24

Light Therapy

Have you ever noticed how great everybody seems to feel when it's a beautiful, sunny day? People are energized, "up," and eager to go out and live it up. In contrast, think of the first day we go back to "standard time." By turning the clocks back an hour, many of us find ourselves still at work after nightfall. That's when everybody starts complaining: "I just hate it when it gets dark so early!" "It's so depressing." "I feel like I should be home in bed."

Light, or the lack of light, probably affects our emotional and physical health even more than most of us realize. It's common knowledge that as the days grow shorter or you go farther north, the rates of depression, suicide, and alcoholism increase markedly. The symptoms of PMS can also become more severe as the days grow shorter and darker. In fact, some women who never get PMS during the rest of the year find themselves really suffering during the winter months. And for those who get PMS regularly, the lack of light can make it even worse.

THE PMS-LIGHT CONNECTION

But why would PMS be connected to light? The answer has to do with metabolic cycles that are, for the most part, light-dependent. Within your body, hundreds of different cycles (involving hunger, temperature, sleep, etc.) play out every day, governed by your very own twenty-four-hour internal clock. One of those cycles, the sleep cycle, is very much affected by the presence and absence of light. When the sun goes down or you find yourself in a dark, dimly lit area, your brain begins to produce a neurotransmitter called *melatonin*, which shifts your body into a "lower gear," makes you feel drowsy, and gets your body ready for sleep. Melatonin is synthesized from another neurotransmitter called *serotonin*, and these two substances can easily be converted from one to the other. For example, when you're exposed to bright light, your brain starts making serotonin. Take away that light, and your body will begin converting serotonin to melatonin. Switch the bright light back on, and the melatonin will start to convert back to serotonin.

Serotonin has the opposite effect of melatonin. It wakes you up, makes you feel alert, energetic, happy, confident, and just plain good. You want to have a plentiful supply of serotonin, not only for its "feel good" effects, but also to provide the raw material for melatonin, so that you can fall asleep at night. Without enough serotonin, you can wind up feeling depressed, aggressive, and irritable, with a fierce craving for sugar and other carbohydrates—the foods that just so happen to increase serotonin levels in the brain. And you can end up with a bad case of insomnia.

If you think the symptoms of too little serotonin and melatonin sound like some of the classic signs of PMS (depression, irritability, aggression, sugar cravings, insomnia), you're right. And guess what? Your melatonin/serotonin levels must *drop* in order for ovulation to occur. That means you're automatically set up for sleep troubles, depression, mood swings, and carbo cravings during the last two weeks of your cycle—your PMS phase.

It seems clear that too little serotonin and melatonin can play a part in bringing on PMS or making it worse. And there's one thing that can markedly decrease your levels of these important neurotransmitters—too little light.

DISRUPTION OF THE MELATONIN/SEROTONIN CYCLE

Since light turns on serotonin production, and darkness turns it off and triggers production of melatonin, you can imagine how messed up your sleep/wake cycle can get when you travel across time lines. Imagine finding yourself in the bright sunlight of Paris at 8:00 A.M., just when your West Coast body is gearing up for an 11:00 P.M. burst of melatonin. Or working the midnight shift and going to bed at 8:00 A.M. with your serotonin production in full swing. No wonder travelers get jet lag that they just can't shake, and graveyard-shift workers get less sleep than just about anybody on the planet. If they're women, they probably get some pretty bad cases of PMS, as well.

Another scenario that really disrupts the serotonin/melatonin cycle is living in an area far to the north, like Alaska, where in winter it may be dark until noon, with darkness falling again at 3:00 P.M. Serotonin manufacture is extremely difficult under these conditions, so it's no wonder that many people in such areas fall into terrible depressions during the winter. They may also find that any existing conditions, like PMS, alcoholism, bipolar disorder, sleep disorders, and bulimia nervosa, become worse at this time. It's not surprising that all of these conditions are related to low serotonin levels.

As you can see, a lack of light and a lack of serotonin are very much related. Take a look at the symptoms caused by too little of either:

- A change in appetite, most notably a craving for sweet or starchy foods
- Difficulty concentrating
- Fatigue

- Fear of social rejection
- Irritability
- Lack of interest in socializing
- Reduced energy levels
- Tendency to oversleep
- Weight gain

All of these symptoms are also seen in PMS, which seems to be at least partially the result of a domino effect: the lack of light causes a lack of serotonin, which causes a worsening of PMS symptoms. The lack of serotonin also results in a lack of melatonin, a condition often seen in those with a severe form of PMS called premenstrual dysphoric disorder (PMDD).

What does this mean to you, the PMS sufferer? Get some light into your life! This may be especially true if you only get PMS during the fall or winter, if depression is a problem, or if you have PMDD. By getting plenty of light, you'll automatically increase not only your serotonin levels but your melatonin levels, as well.

HOW LIGHT THERAPY WORKS

To increase your serotonin production, you'll need exposure to either full-spectrum light (the kind we get from the sun) or a bright white light. (The incandescent lights that most of us have in our lamps just don't work.) If you live in a sunny area, undergoing light therapy is easy. Just take a walk in the bright sunlight for about ten minutes each day, preferably in the early morning. Don't wear sunglasses or tinted contacts, so your eyes will be exposed to the light rays. (Yet don't look directly at the sun.) If you live in a non-sunny area, try changing your light bulbs from incandescent to full-spectrum bulbs to see if that makes a difference.

If you feel you need something stronger, you may want to purchase a special light box that can provide fluorescent full-spectrum light (the same as natural daylight without UV emissions) or a bright white light that contains no UV wavelengths. (UV can cause skin cancer.) There are also new systems that use cool-white, triphosphor, and bi-axial lamps. What's most important is that the level of light produced by the box matches the light you'd find outdoors either right after sunrise or right before sunset.

The light is measured in units called *lux*, and the typical light box provides 10,000 lux. Daylight is about 5,000 lux and it takes at least 2,500 lux to have a therapeutic effect on the body's internal clock.

USING THE LIGHT BOX

To use the light box, turn it on and sit in front of it once a day during the fall and winter seasons. Don't look directly at the light, but face the box. The average length of a session is between fifteen and forty-five minutes, during which you can read, eat, or do whatever you want while receiving light therapy. Just don't close your eyes or wear tinted glasses or tinted contacts.

Most people schedule their light therapy sessions during the morning, before 10:00 A.M. But if you feel extremely dragged out and sleepy when the alarm goes off in the morning, you may need to get your light therapy *first thing* in the morning (before 8:00 A.M.). That's becaue feeling super-groggy in the morning may be a sign that your melatonin levels are still flying high, even though they should be receding by that hour. Eight out of ten people who have a severe form of depression called seasonal affective disorder (SAD) have melatonin levels that peak at wake-up time. By taking light therapy early in the morning, you can decrease your melatonin levels, while simultaneously pumping up your levels of the "wake-up" hormone serotonin.

On the other hand, if your problem is waking up in the middle of the night and not being able to fall asleep again, your melatonin levels may be receding too soon. In that case, try light therapy in the evening.

WARNING: The side effects of light therapy are minimal and usually the result of overdoing it. But if you experience eye redness, eyestrain, fatigue, headaches, irritability, or an inability to sleep (usually due to evening light therapy), either limit your exposure or terminate the therapy. If your skin or eyes are sensitive to light, or if you're taking antibiotics, antipsychotic drugs, or medication for psoriasis or vitiligo, be sure to consult your doctor before using light therapy.

WHERE CAN I FIND A LIGHT BOX?

You can do light therapy by yourself, without the help of a practitioner. But it's always best to see a medical doctor for advice about how to use light therapy, and/or to get a complete examination if you're experiencing severe depression. You can find a selection of light boxes from a company called Light for Health, 942 Twisted Oak Lane, Buffalo Grove, IL 60089; phone: (800) 468-1104; E-mail: info@lightforhealth.com; website: www.lightforhealth.com. Prices range from about $350–$500, but some insurance companies cover at least part of the cost if the light box is prescribed by a doctor.

25

Sleep

Just about any condition can be improved by a good night's sleep—and, conversely, can be made worse by a lousy night's sleep. If you're not getting enough sleep, you can find yourself depressed, tired, irritable, distracted, moody, suffering from headaches, and just plain "off." Hey, that sounds a lot like the symptoms of both PMS and a lack of serotonin! And it just so happens that you're *less* likely to get the sleep you need during the PMS phase because your melatonin/serotonin levels will drop just before ovulation. (See Chapter 24 for a complete explanation.) Because of this, you can easily find yourself caught in a vicious circle—PMS causes sleep problems and too little sleep exacerbates PMS.

Clearly, the last thing you need when you've got PMS is insomnia. So it's imperative that you do whatever you can to get a full measure of good-quality sleep every single night. How do you do that? One important way is to cultivate both the production and preservation of your serotonin levels.

SEROTONIN FOR SLEEP

As discussed in Chapter 24, two major neurotransmitters govern the sleep cycle—serotonin and melatonin. If your serotonin levels are high, you'll most likely feel calm, happy, and satisfied. Then, when dark falls, your high levels of serotonin will be converted to melatonin, and you'll sleep like a baby. In the morning, when dawn's early light strikes your eyes, the melatonin will convert back to serotonin and you'll wake up feeling like a million bucks.

Unfortunately, all bets are off if you're lacking in serotonin/melatonin. And if you've got PMS, chances are good that you are lacking in these important neurotransmitters, setting the stage for difficulty falling asleep, poor-quality sleep, and middle of the night awakenings. So it's crucial that you boost and preserve your precious serotonin levels if you want to get enough sleep. (If you've got plenty of serotonin, you'll automatically have plenty of its converted version, melatonin.)

THE SEROTONIN BOOSTERS

Luckily, even if nature is depriving you of your share of serotonin, you can do plenty to increase your levels of this important substance in other ways. Try these:

• **Increase your tryptophan supply**—Serotonin and, by extension, melatonin are manufactured within your body from the essential amino acid *tryptophan*. It's called an "essential" amino acid because your body can't manufacture tryptophan on its own, so you need to get it from the foods you eat. Luckily, that's easy since tryptophan is found in lots of different foods, most notably turkey, milk, eggs, cheese, fish, soybeans, and potatoes. So a light bedtime snack of a tryptophan-rich food (e.g., a glass of warm milk or a slice of turkey) may be just what's needed to pack you off to dreamland. You can also take tryptophan supplements in the form of 5-hydroxy-tryptophan, which is available at health-food stores.

- **Increase carbohydrate consumption**—Getting plenty of tryptophan is a good start, but that alone won't necessarily do the trick. That's because tryptophan needs to get into your brain before it can be converted to the good stuff, serotonin. And to do that, it must cross the *blood/brain barrier*, a filter that's designed to keep out bacteria, viruses, and other toxins that can attack your brain. Unfortunately, tryptophan has a hard time blasting through this barrier, and often needs a little something extra to speed its passage. Help can be found in the form of carbohydrates. Carbos spur the release of insulin, and when insulin rushes into the brain, tryptophan tags along for the ride. So, when you start getting sugar cravings during your PMS phase, it may be your body's way of getting extra tryptophan into your brain where it can be made into serotonin. So consider adding a couple of crackers or a slice of toast to your tryptophan-rich bedtime snack to ensure a good night's sleep.

- **Take vitamin B$_6$**—Okay, so you've eaten plenty of tryptophan-containing foods and plenty of carbohydrates to get the tryptophan into your brain. Are you home free? Not necessarily. That's because Vitamin B$_6$ is needed to carry out the conversion from tryptophan to serotonin. If you're lacking in B$_6$, your serotonin levels may stay low, no matter what you're eating. Try taking at least 50 mg of B$_6$ throughout the month, and increase the dose slightly just before menstruation.

- **Don't restrict sodium too drastically**—I know, I know! I've already told you to "shun salt" in order to ease water retention. But if you cut back too much, you may unwittingly decrease your serotonin supply, since sodium helps keep serotonin active within the cell. As with most things, moderation is the key. Taking in 3 to 4 grams of sodium per day should be adequate for maintaining serotonin, without promoting water retention.

- **Get plenty of exposure to light**—As discussed in Chapter 24, light is necessary for serotonin production, and if you don't get enough of it, you're probably making lesser amounts of serotonin/melatonin. Get some early-morning light every day, or consider buying a light box.

• **Take niacinamide**—Tryptophan is the raw material for two things inside the body: serotonin and niacinamide, a form of the vitamin niacin. If you take plenty of niacinamide in supplement form, your body can then concentrate on producing serotonin. Conversely, if you've got low levels of niacinamide, some of your tryptophan will be used up making more of this vitamin. Niacin doesn't have the same effect on serotonin levels, so be sure to take it in the form of niacinamide. A daily dose of 50 mg should be sufficient.

You can also skip the whole serotonin conversion process and get to the heart of the matter—increasing your melatonin supply—by taking melatonin in supplement form. Many people who have trouble falling asleep have been helped by taking nightly doses of between 1 and 3 mg of melatonin. Taking more than 3 mg may actually induce insomnia, so don't assume that more is better. And don't take melatonin if you're pregnant, nursing, trying to conceive, taking steroids or MAO inhibitors, or if you have a compromised immune system.

GOOD SLEEP HABITS

No chapter on sleep would be complete without at least a quick rundown of basic habits that contribute to good sleep. To regulate your sleeping schedule and make sure you get plenty of good-quality sleep, consider the following guidelines:

• **Determine the amount of sleep you need**—Eight hours may not be enough—or it may be too much! (It's possible that you're trying to force yourself to get more sleep than you really need.) Everybody's different, so experiment to find out how many hours you need in order to feel alert, refreshed, and rested. Then, arrange your schedule to make sure you get that amount.

- **Get up and go to bed at the same time every day**—Just about everybody likes the idea of sleeping in on the weekends. But if you get up an hour or two later on the weekends, your "internal clock" will be thrown off. Then, when bedtime rolls around, you may find yourself unable to fall asleep. Try to keep the same sleeping schedule, even on weekends.

- **Make sure your mattress and pillow are comfortable**—You need the right amount of support from your mattress and pillow, coupled with the right amount of cushioning. What's the "right amount"? Only you can make that decision. If a stiff neck bothers you during the night or you wake up with a sore back, something's wrong. Experiment to find the pillow, mattress, and mattress cover that feel best to you.

- **Block out noise and light**—The sounds of traffic, dogs barking, kids playing, or machinery blasting can ruin an otherwise good night's sleep. A fan or white noise machine creates steady background noise that can muffle disturbing sounds. Another sleep-killer is light. If you've got a street lamp shining through your window or your room is too light overall, melatonin production can be impaired, making it difficult for you to fall asleep. Try heavy drapes or blackout shades to make your bedroom as dark as possible.

- **Keep it cool, but not cold**—If you feel either hot or cold, you may have trouble sleeping. Try to keep your bedroom between fifty-five and sixty-five degrees, but keep a warm blanket on hand.

- **Use your bed only for sleeping and sex**—Eating, playing with your kids, writing letters, watching TV, doing office work—what *don't* we do in bed? Because of that, our beds can become associated with activity rather than rest. But if you keep your bed sacred, making it a place that you use only for sleeping and sex, your mind and body will automatically shift into the relaxation/sleep mode when you get into bed.

- **Wind down for about an hour before retiring**—Running around, doing chores, watching a scary movie, paying bills, or fighting with your husband are not preludes to a good night's sleep. Yet many of us are busy, busy, busy until we fall into bed, exhausted. Then, surprise! We can't seem to fall asleep. Decelerate before you attempt to drift into dreamland. Try taking a nice long bath, doing yoga, engaging in quiet conversation, making love, doing progressive relaxation exercises, or anything else that can help you wind down before it's time to go to sleep.

• **Don't drink alcohol before bedtime**—As you know, alcohol is a no-no for PMS sufferers anyway, but it's double trouble for problem sleepers. Besides disrupting normal sleep patterns, alcohol can trigger headaches and become habit-forming, so don't attempt to induce sleep this way.

• **Don't eat a heavy meal or drink a lot of liquid before bedtime**—A light bedtime snack can help you sleep, but forcing your body to digest a heavy meal while you're lying down can keep you awake. And, of course, drinking too much liquid before retiring will result in sleep-disrupting middle-of-the-night trips to the bathroom.

• **Stay away from caffeine**—Here's another no-no for PMS, especially before bedtime. The caffeine found in coffee, black tea, soda, chocolate, and cocoa is a stimulant that makes it difficult to fall asleep and stay asleep.

• **If you nap, do so with caution**—Napping can upset your sleeping schedule, especially if you nap for more than an hour. If you really feel exhausted, take a short nap (one hour or less) in the afternoon. Don't nap in the morning or evening, since it's too close to wake-up time or bedtime. Remember that feeling tired at the end of the day is a *good* thing—it should help you fall asleep.

• **If you can't sleep, get up**—If you've been lying in bed for more than one-half hour with no luck, get up and do something monotonous, like folding laundry. You can read, if you want, but make sure you're sitting up—and don't do it in bed. Then, when you feel really tired, go back to bed and try again. If you still can't sleep, repeat the process. The idea is to associate your bed with sleep—not wakefulness.

AND IF THAT DOESN'T HELP . . .

As a sometime insomniac myself, I find that I can't finish this chapter without revealing every last little sleeping trick I've discovered. One is magnesium, nature's very own tranquilizer. You can take a 200 mg or 400 mg tablet along with your cup of warm milk before bedtime and your carbo snack. Then, for good measure, throw in a couple of valerian tablets, to relax you further. And, if you take progesterone, save it for bedtime because it, too, has a nice tranquilizing effect. Some people have good luck with melatonin supplements (take 1–3 mg, but not more). Oh, and if your partner's snoring bothers you, get up and go sleep in another room (if possible).

And should you have a night when *nothing* seems to work (and I've had them, believe me!), try to keep things in perspective and stay calm. Getting worried and upset about your insomnia will almost certainly ruin any possibility of falling asleep. So relax. Even if you pull an all-nighter, at the very worst you'll feel tired and dragged out the next day—not exactly a life-threatening situation. And chances are wonderful that you'll sleep like a log the following night!

Afterword

When I was a teenager, the big menstrual difficulty that everybody talked about was cramps. And, according to the girls in my neighborhood, there was only one cure: a spoonful of Karo syrup! These were also the days when we were told, "It's all in your mind. Just forget about it and it'll go away." What a long way we've come! Today we understand a great deal about the etiology of PMS and we can now do many things to ease our discomfort and distress. Most, if not all, of them are right here in this book.

But as I thumbed through the pages of the finished manuscript, an odd thought struck me. Almost every one of the "25 Natural Ways To Relieve PMS" could also benefit men, non-PMS women, and children! That's because they support the basic principles of good health. And although there are complex reasons why diet, exercise, relaxation, stress reduction, "good" fats, positive thinking, light, and sleep can all ease the symptoms of PMS, the truth is these things are good for you no matter what. Which brings me to this conclusion: *The best way to fight PMS is to build your health to epic proportions*. And isn't that the answer to just about any physical problem?

I send you my very best wishes on your quest to banish PMS from your life. May you find health, happiness, and sanity—every day of the month!

Index